Homemade Hand Sanitizer & Face Mask

Homemade Hand Sanitizer

Table of Contents

INTRODUCTION 1

ABOUT THIS GUIDE 3

DIY HOMEMADE HAND SANITIZER ALCOHOL FREE.4

    WHY USE ALCOHOL AS A BASE RATHER THAN WITCH HAZEL? 5
    WHY TO MAKE YOUR OWN HAND SANITIZER? 6
    WHAT TO STORE YOUR HAND SANITIZER IN? 7
    WHAT ESSENTIAL OILS ARE BEST FOR HOMEMADE HAND SANITIZER? 7
    STEPS 8

DIY HAND SANITIZER SPRAY {ALCOHOL-FREE AND KID-SAFE} 12

    HAND SANITIZER SHOULD NOT REPLACE HAND WASHING 14
    STEPS 15

DIY HAND SANITIZER WITH ALCOHOL 20

    ARE HAND SANITIZERS EFFECTIVE AND ANTIVIRAL? 21
    WHAT INGREDIENTS DO YOU NEED TO MAKE HAND SANITIZER? 23
    WHAT ELSE DO YOU NEED TO MAKE HAND SANITIZER? 25
    STEPS 25

DIY HAND SANITIZER WITH ALCOHOL {FRESH ALOE VERA + VODKA} 29

    HOW TO CUT FRESH ALOE 30
    STEPS 36

METHOD 1: DIY DISINFECTING WIPES (NATURAL & REUSABLE) 45

- Undisclosed ingredients in commercial disinfecting wipes 46
- Top antibacterial essential oils for homemade cleaning wipes 47
- Ingredients for DIY disinfecting wipes 49
- Save money on cleaning wipes with reusable cloths 51
- How to use these sanitizing wipes 52
- Steps 53

METHOD 2: DIY SANITIZER WIPES AT HOME 59

- What ingredients work for disinfectant wipes? 59
- How can I make disinfectant wipes with bleach? 61
- How can I make disinfectant wipes without bleach? 62
- What surfaces in my home are safe to clean with disinfectant wipes? 62
- What else should I remember when using disinfectant wipes? 63
- Tips 64
- Is It Safe to Use Vodka as Hand Sanitizer? 65

Introduction

Hand sanitizer is a fluid, spray, or gel widely used on hands to decrease viruses and bacteria. Handwashing with soap and water is usually preferred in most environments and it cannot extract harmful chemicals unlike soap and water. People can wipe away the hand sanitizer incorrectly before it has been dried, and some are quite useful because the concentrations of alcohol are too low.

Hand sanitizers based on alcohol are superior in most health-care environments to hand washing with soap and water. Reasons include being treated better and being more effective. Hand washing with soap and water only can be done if contamination can be observed, or after use of the toilet, it should be done.

Usually, alcohol-based versions contain a mixture of isopropyl alcohol, ethanol (ethyl alcohol), or n-propanol, with the most effective versions containing 60 to 95 per cent alcohol. Care should be taken because it is flame-retardant. Hand sanitizer based with alcohol protects against a large variety of microorganisms but not spores. Compounds like glycerol can be added to avoid skin drying. Many variants contain fragrances; however, due to the possibility of allergic reactions these are discouraged. Non-alcoholic versions typically contain benzalkonium chloride or triclosan; however, they are less effective than alcoholic versions.

About This Guide

This guide is all about the Homemade Hand Sanitizer and it is unique from all of the others. The way the guideline is designed makes it easier to find the solution you are looking for. Go ahead and click the Guide to see for yourself. Nice bold headings direct your eyes to only the section you like, and you do not have to read the whole text for a quick response. This guide offers an exhaustive description of all facets of DIY your Hand Sanitizer at home. Need details about how to get started? Here is the description too. So, place this tutorial up on your bookcase in a prominent spot. We are confident you will go back to that again and again.

DIY Homemade Hand Sanitizer Alcohol Free

This Homemade Hand Sanitizer is incredibly cheap and easy to make and also non-toxic!

Important Note: Prior using a home remedy, every time supervision of a health care provider is necessary, as this has never been checked in a laboratory. Also, this hand sanitizer formulation does not have the sixty percent + alcohol level required by the CDC and other medical associations for hand sanitizer to combat against virus effectively.

Everybody has never been a hand sanitizer fan; you know the common kind all around dispensers! someone has had delicate skin and they just don't comply with them. In reality, whenever someone has had to use these, their skin fissures, and bleeds everywhere within hours. And when they took a course on food standards, they told us that proper usage and methods of hand washing are much more productive.

How to make hand sanitizer without alcohol?

You should use Witch Hazel instead of alcohol as the basis and is better for fighting off germs. It might not be as strong as Vodka claims, but it does some good! Moreover, many individuals who choose to use a handmade hand sanitizer for kids tend to use Witch Hazel as a basis instead of alcohol. You might also want to check out the plant therapy blend of Germ Buster Essential Oils which is designed for babies. Not all the essential oils are mostly safe for kids, so it's nice to have a mixture made up already.

Why use alcohol as a base rather than Witch Hazel?

In destroying most germs, alcohol such as isopropyl (rubbing alcohol) is very efficient. Witch hazel is productive but not so much. Research says that 60-90% of alcohol is safer, which seems fairly decent. Particularly when you're talking about moving from the plane to the rental cars.

Why to make your own hand sanitizer?

It's non-toxic There are some strong brands to be purchased in quality food shops on the market. But the regular grocery store products are replete with harmful chemicals.

Cost – Making your own hand sanitizer is very economically viable, and also super easy. We can produce a batch in just a few minutes lasting for months.

Sensitive skin – Those who have very sensitive skin, so the sanitizer must be made by considering the sensitivity of the skin.

Traveling – That kind of never even needs a description! It's super convenient and have something to destroy off germs even when you are travelling.

Cold and flu season – Although alcohol is not 100 percent efficient for all pathogens, isopropyl alcohol is 99.9% successful for non-spore - forming bacteria and combats several other viruses and seasonal flu.

What to store your hand sanitizer in?

Any squeeze or little bottle of spray that you have. The 2 you see pictured here used to be store hand sanitizer bottles. In shops you can also verify the trip bottle category, while these types of bottles are not as excellent quality and will be leaked over time. REI also has a great selection of small containers that are useful for homemade bath & body brands to start taking backpacking.

Try using an opaque dark colored bottle to protect essential oils, if you can spot one, (they are prone to light). Obviously, you have not to be concerned a lot about this, because these hand sanitizer bottles can remain in a dark for long.

What essential oils are best for homemade hand sanitizer?

Lemon essential oil - Antiseptic properties, disinfectants, and antifungals.

Lavender essential oil - Anti-bacterial, antiviral, and I also love that smell!

Tea Tree essential oil – Anti-fungal, antimicrobial, antiseptic, antiviral, and antibacterial – whew... that's a lot!

Others to consider – There are also antibacterial effects of eucalyptus, clove, cinnamon, lime, peppermint, rosemary, herb, and garlic.

Steps

An easy way to use non-toxic hand sanitizer suitable for both traveling and running errands!

INGREDIENTS

For a spray bottle:

- 3 Tablespoons Aloe Vera gel
- 3 Tablespoons witch hazel, isopropyl alcohol, ethanol, or vodka
- 15 drops lemon essential oil
- 15 drops lavender essential oil
- 15-30 drops of tea tree essential oil, see notes

For a squeeze bottle:

- 1/4 cup Aloe Vera gel

- 2 Tablespoons witch hazel, isopropyl alcohol, ethanol, or vodka
- 15 drops lemon essential oil
- 15 drops lavender essential oil
- 15-30 drops of tea tree essential oil, see notes

INSTRUCTIONS

1. Mix all the ingredients together either for the recycle spray or squeeze bottle. You can do this by bringing them specifically into your tank through a funnel. Or you can blend them together in a small pot, then drain them into your selected jar (or very cautiously).

2. If you are using a glass bottle, make sure to keep it in a dark position to better protect the essential oils' qualities. Essential oils can segregate over time, and before every use, you must shake up your hand sanitizer.

NOTES

The more oil you use for tea tree, the more efficient it is in preventing infections. Honestly, however, someone have some intolerances to this specific oil, so use the minimal quantity that appears to work great for skin. These are often commonly considered to be healthy oils for most users, as an essential oil safeguard. However, bear in mind that they do not work for you and if you have any effects at all, you can still receive advice from a health practitioner / abandon using them! In certain cases, any of these oils can also have a photosensitivity where you will get a discomfort when the skin is exposed to the light.

DIY Hand Sanitizer Spray {Alcohol-free and Kid-Safe}

Everyone must start making their own DIY items because we are all worried about common toxics. Since these collect in our bodies, everybody's chief concern is toxic chemicals and endocrine disruptors, and they have been associated with all kinds of ailments alongside cancer. It makes you question if all of the cancer that surrounds us is relevant to everything, we 're prone to.

We have to make it a mission to reduce our children's exposure to toxic chemicals, and one of the best ways to do so when you make your own DIY products. That way, you know exactly what's in everything. For this we have to know that the ingredients are clean, and we don't have to use preservatives because we have to make them in small quantities.

Hand sanitizer is one of the items we have to keep in our diaper bag. Ideally, we 'd always clean our hands with proper soap and water but that isn't always possible, and this is where hand sanitizer fits in.

What's wrong with hand sanitizers?

Some sanitizers have additives which we have to avoid within our family. Here are the major concerns:

Triclosan: Is used in cosmetic products as bactericide. The concern with this is it helps to create antibiotic resistant bacteria and has been related to degradation of hormone activity.

Fragrances: The issue with this is that corporations are not forced to reveal what is in their scents and much of the time the chemicals used to make them include phthalates and parabens-both endocrine disruptors.

Alcohol: This is one of the most essential components in hand sanitizer and the logic they smell the way they do. The trouble with that is that it might be dangerous for them if your child were to consume it – and things like that happened. As for other kinds of alcohols being used hand sanitizers, there are several other questions too.

Hand sanitizer should NOT replace hand washing

This may sound like rational thinking, but hand sanitizers should be used only when there is no water and soap. You can simply make your own DIY hand sanitizer that's safe and efficacious at residence, and then use whenever you're out there.

In my particular instance, you will find yourself in need of daily use of the hand sanitizer. when there's no water and soap approximately, children mostly would like to snack, and once they snack, we might have a snack too. So, that's one of those factors we have to carry with us always.

Methods for this hand sanitizer do not contain alcohol because we don't want to use alcohol on our children. In this method the microbe-killing components are the essential oils. If you want not to use essential oils, you will need to change this formula to use at least 60 per cent of alcohol mixing.

Tip to keep your home disinfected:

If you're searching for a house sanitizer, our go-to is Nature Energy, it's just as good as bleach but without the harmful chemicals. Force of Nature is registered as EPA for the disinfection and sanitization of health facilities, ICUs, daycares, educational institutions and more.

DIY Hand Sanitizer Spray:

This method makes this one-ounce spray bottle sufficient to fill up. If you reuse an old bottle of hand sanitizer, you'll definitely need 2 oz of this method so just almost double product. Bear in mind that this recycle does not comprise additives so you should make or use it in small lots.

The recipes are made in about 1 minute.

Steps

INGREDIENTS

- 1 oz glass spray bottle

- 1 tablespoon Aloe Vera spray or Aloe Vera gel (after making this recipe many times, I recommend using the Aloe Vera spray)
- 1 tablespoon alcohol-free witch hazel
- ¼ teaspoon vitamin E oil
- 30-36 drops of Germ Destroyer (get on Amazon)
- If you don't have Germ Destroyer, you can use 30 drops to tea tree oil and 5-10 drops of lavender essential oil

INSTRUCTIONS

This is such a simple recipe to make!

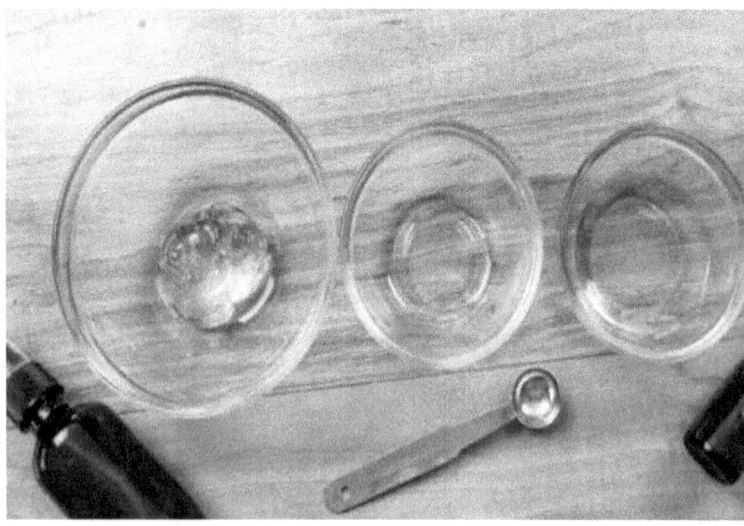

1. If you are using the Aloe Vera moisturizer, all you have to do is use a small funnel to put all the additives into the bottle. Then shake it and it's prepared.

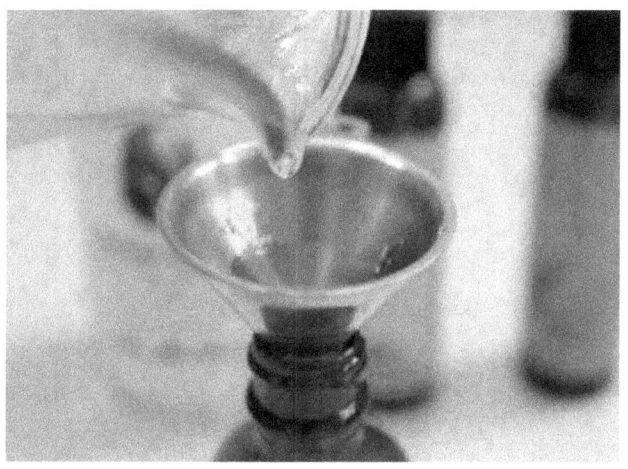

2. If you use Aloe Vera gel though, then you'll have to blend all the additives in a small glass jar.

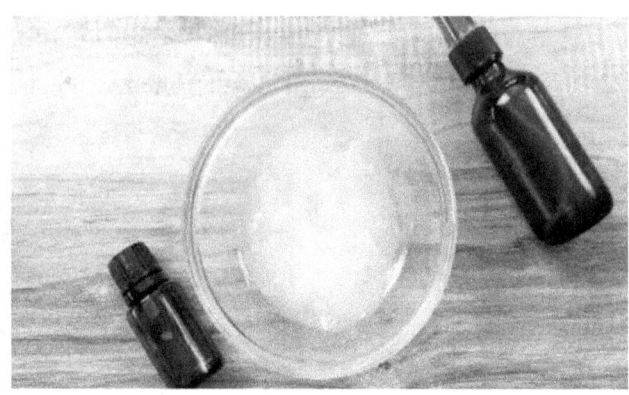

3. Mix them together well so that the gel coherence has become more liquid.
4. Move into the flask. Using a pipette, it is simple to pour it if you used the gel.

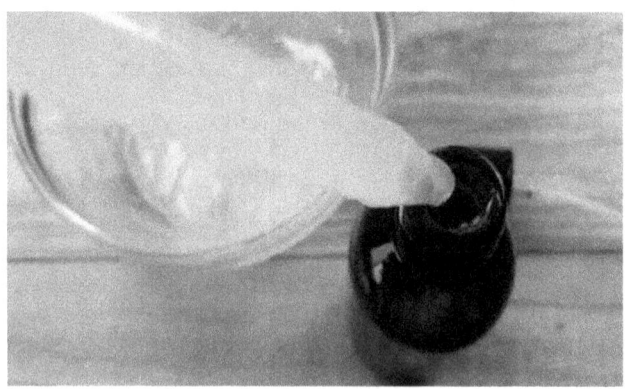

5. Giving it shake, and it is prepared! Spray as you would any standard hand sanitizer spray on your hands.

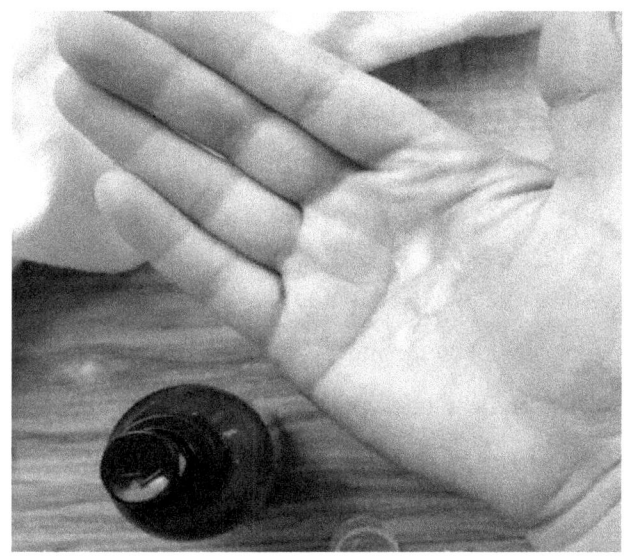

6. Keep it in your bag and use it, as necessary. Before any use do not hesitate to shake it. You will absolutely adore this recipe.

DIY Hand Sanitizer With Alcohol

As the virus pandemic started to expand, wherever feasible the Centers for Disease Control has suggested "social distancing" and self-isolation. And one consequence of that, as you may have realized, is things flying off the shelves at your local supermarket. One of those stuff? Hand sanitizer.

Remember what everybody is going to buy next — alcohol, aloe vera, and essential oils — and get ahead of the trend while you're going to stock up on non-perishables, drugs, and other vital things you may need in the next several weeks.

No, that's not the remedy for a trendy, boozy beverage, if you like, a quarantine. As individuals (namely, Googling) figure out how to make their own home sanitizer — know, hand sanitizer was the first thing people came after during the first virus initial attack! — Isopropyl alcohol, aloe Vera gel and essential oils are expected to be the next priorities for the communities. If you've been looking for DIY hand sanitizers, here's what you'd like to know — from theories to reality, to the advice of a specialist on how to make it yourself.

Are hand sanitizers effective and antiviral?

Next, it's absolutely justifiable that you want to know if it's successful before you go through the hassle of learning to make hand sanitizer at home. And perhaps most significantly if the virus is successful.

The Centers for Disease Control suggested ethanol-based (alcohol-based) sanitizers such as hand sanitizers as a means of preventing the transmission of virus in an official comment entitled, "CDC Report for Healthcare Workers on Hand Hygiene during the Reaction to the Global resurgence of virus."

"CDC guidelines illustrate the essential role of hygiene practices in avoiding pathogens from spreading to a wide variety of pathogens in healthcare settings," the statement says. "The potential of hand hygiene, especially hand washing or the use of hand sanitizers dependent on alcohol to deter infections, is linked to decreases in the number of active microbes that peripherally contaminate the hands."

"Hand washing manually extracts contaminants although laboratory results indicate that 60 percent ethanol and 70 percent isopropanol, the active ingredients in CDC-recommended alcohol-based hand sanitizers, detoxify biologically-related viruses with identical physical characteristics to the 2019-virus," it adds.

The CDC has also suggested hand sanitizers dependent on alcohol as the "preferred method of hygiene practices in healthcare environments."

You would like to ensure you have 99 percent isopropyl or rubbing alcohol, Aloe Vera jelly, and essential oils such as tea tree oil, lavender, citrus, clove, peppermint, frankincense, thyme and/or oregano oil, if you'd like to make it at home.

Nevertheless, it is important to keep in mind that antibacterial is not the same as antiviral. Since the virus came into being, this may not be as good for other essential oils including antibacterial properties.

These all have antibacterial properties so I would suggest them. "Just note, this virus cannot function the same as other antibacterial agents." So, to be sure, while DIY home sanitizer is not suggested as a 100 percent security feature, here is the break down if you should try to make it.

What ingredients do you need to make hand sanitizer?

Hand sanitizer with three primary components can indeed be made at home: isopropyl alcohol (ninety-one per cent or higher), Aloe Vera powder, and maybe a few drops of essential oil. Now, until you mix all those items, there are some points you should learn.

Isopropyl alcohol is the principal sanitizing component in this recipe for DIY hand sanitizer. To keep your at-home sanitizer as safe as possible, keep sure you substitute alcohol that is up to or above ninety-one per cent alcohol. Optimally, the most you can achieve is ninety nine percent, but anything over 91 would also work well to dispose of bacteria and viruses.

Aloe Vera gel is available in most of the markets. Put it another way, if you have an Aloe Vera plant, you should break off a plant leaf and use it to cure (and sanitize) as its properties. Because of its moisturizing qualities it is also essential to the recipe; it prevents the skin from drying out. The alcohol in this manual sanitizer method will cause your skin to dry out without Aloe Vera.

There are some which you can use for sanitizer when it relates to essential oils. Though, tea tree is probably the most popular basic oil to be used for sanitizer. Tea tree oil has antibacterial effects as well as antiviral, antifungal and anti-inflammatory properties. Although work on whether the essential oil of the tea tree virus can effectively protect is minimal, it is assumed to fend off the microbes involved with acne, staphylococci, micrococci, Enterococcus faecalis and Pseudomonas aeruginosa.

Cinnamon is another basic oil that is suggested for producing a hand sanitizer. In certain species, cinnamon essentially "deactivated" the viral constituents.

If you're only trying to feel nice in your hand sanitizer, try using lemon, citrus, peppermint, or lavender. That essential oil you choose, 8-15 drops should do the method everywhere.

What else do you need to make hand sanitizer?

Among these three primary components, you'll also need a mixing pot, spoon, measuring cup and a funnel. Though these items are not essential, they definitely make the procedures of weighing and sanitation much simpler!

Steps

How to make DIY hand sanitizer

All is the ratio. The ratio that you need to the most powerful hand sanitizer relies on how much alcohol you consume.

For e.g., if you're using ninety-one per cent Isopropyl alcohol, you're going to want a 3:2 ratio, 3 tablespoons of alcohol to Aloe teaspoons. When you use ninety-nine per cent isopropyl alcohol, you're going to want a ratio of 2:1 (3 T alcohol, 1.5 T alcohol).

If you use ninety-one per cent of Isopropyl alcohol, toss 1 cup into a bowl and mix. Last, apply Aloe Vera gel 2/3 cup. Insert 8-15 drops of the essential oil of your choosing anywhere you want. Bring all together with a spoon, then use a funnel to turn the blend into a filled container.

If you're not using a bottle with a pump, you should insert your DIY hand sanitizer into a travel go-tube and one of those small salad dressing valves that you place in the meals for babies!

Alternatively, a spray bottle will work, too.

- 1 cup Ever clear
- 1/3 cup Aloe Vera
- 2 tablespoons of coconut oil
- A few drops of essential oil
- Hydrogen Peroxide (amount dependent on supply)
- Mix it up in a bowl and portion into a container.

What if I don't have Aloe Vera gel?

No problems, without the Aloe Vera gel you can still make a hand sanitizer. Only swap Aloe Vera with witch hazel. When you use the witch hazel as an option, the sanitizer's quality would feel more like a mist. A spray bottle is probably much better, for that reason.

When you're nervous about washing your hands because of the alcohol, you should add 1/4 teaspoon of vitamin E spray, too.

How else to disinfect at home?

Thorough maintenance is one of the most effective measures that we can do to suppress the virus to avoid it spreading. This involves handwashing but also daily sanitization of our homes.

We should be disinfecting our house periodically as per CDC guidelines. "First and foremost, more than 20 seconds of repeated hand-washing is necessary. Using latex gloves, then wash disinfectant or soap and water surfaces clean. You have to wipe down of chairs, doorknobs, lamp switches, countertops, handles, seats, telephones, buttons, toilets, and sinks.

So, what's the most effective way to wipe down these surfaces?

You can also use 70 percent of alcohol to thoroughly clean surface areas. "You can use 5 T bleach and 1 gallon of water to produce bleach solution. Personally, if you have no alcohol or bleach, you will not consider doing anything to disinfect with any vinegar or baking soda.

After all, the most effective avoidance strategy of all may be simply social distancing.

The distancing from society is quite necessary. It's vitally important that everyone bear this in mind and pay attention. "And our new health care system won't afford the effect of being ill at once... The reason we're doing this is we won avoid the transmission of the epidemic and ease the pressure on our new health care system."

DIY Hand Sanitizer With Alcohol {Fresh Aloe Vera + Vodka}

Store shelves nationwide are cleaned out of hand sanitizer and basic ingredients for DIY models using Isopropyl alcohol, Everclear, and Aloe Vera/487 gel will be nowhere in sight- what to do? Here is another treatment that combines new Aloe Vera and any high-proof alcohol you can obtain.

This recipe is supposed to help those people who have no access to hand sanitizer, isopropyl alcohol, or Everclear. Most shops in city do sell aloe vera gel. A mist hand sanitizer-not a water sanitizer-is this formula.

It seems that many of us just want to know even at this moment we 're vigilant about our own wellbeing and self-care — this recipe is here to

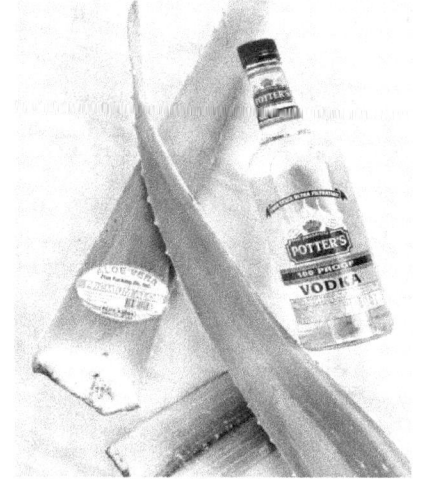

help to give us comfort, a sense of purpose and some germ-busting strength at a period when supplies are momentarily restricted!

This fresh Aloe Vera hand sanitizer has the quality of a fine, sprayable fluid, not a gel!

HOW TO CUT FRESH ALOE

At most food products markets, Mexican markets, and restaurant supplies shops, a spear of new Aloe Vera is widely available for purchase. One stake of Aloe Vera yields around 1 cup of Aloe Vera gel and will remain in the fridge for 1-2 weeks: in the refrigerator for up to 3 months.

When you have ever fileted a fresh tuna, you'll be acquainted with the method of having fresh aloe. To begin with, fresh aloe can be gritty, slimy, and exotic - you'll certainly want a large cutting table and a good knife. I considered a compact knife to be best to use, because you can operate with a sawing action.

Start at the aloe staple core which is the largest portion and also has a white or light color. Check for where the light shading will vanish and resume the green coloring and chop off the white section. Your initial look at the fresh, strange-looking Aloe Vera powder, isn't it?!

Now switch to the Aloe Vera's top and thinnest section. The gel in the slim tip is available, with a limited amount of gel that require just more effort and maneuvering with the knife. Check for a location where the spear is roughly 1 "thick and cut. There may be a certain yellow sap dripping from the Aloe Vera. There can be a stinky scent, too. It's usual!

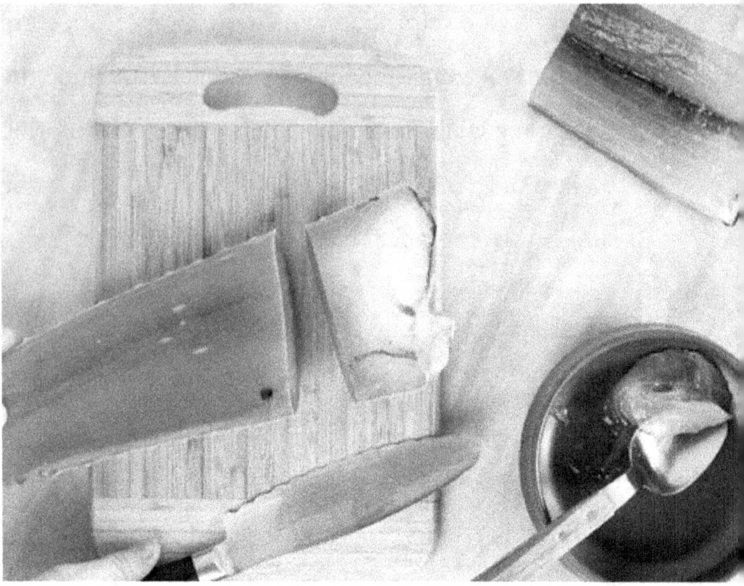

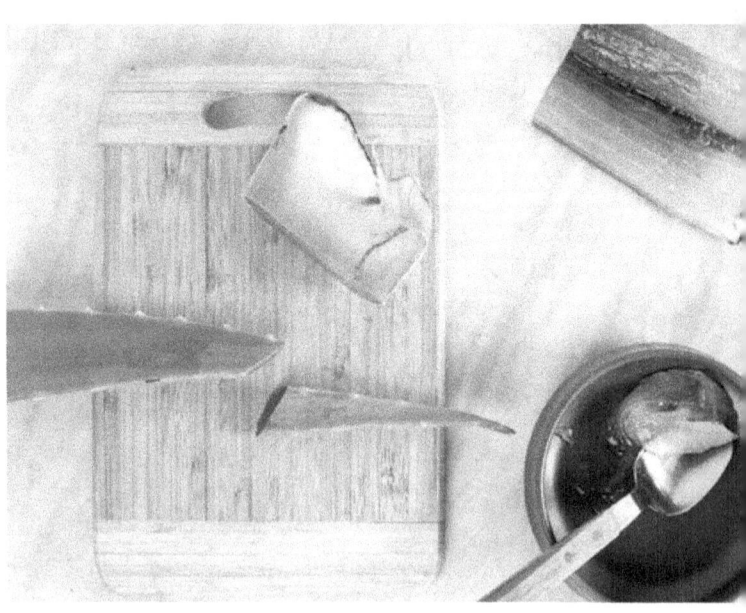

Now you'll be left with an aloe filet comprising of the plant's densest and most flavorful part — Here's how to get to the great stuff!

Switch the aloe on its side for a correlational view, starting from the bottom and largest end of the aloe. Position your knife as near to the edge as feasible, just below the outer green surface, and apply pressure or a soft stitching motion to hold the cut shallow. You can detach your knife after you've managed to make one slice and start softly peeling back the outer green skin. Proceed slicing as nearly as possible to the edge of the aloe filet and peel off the green skin unless you have revealed one part of the aloe entirely.

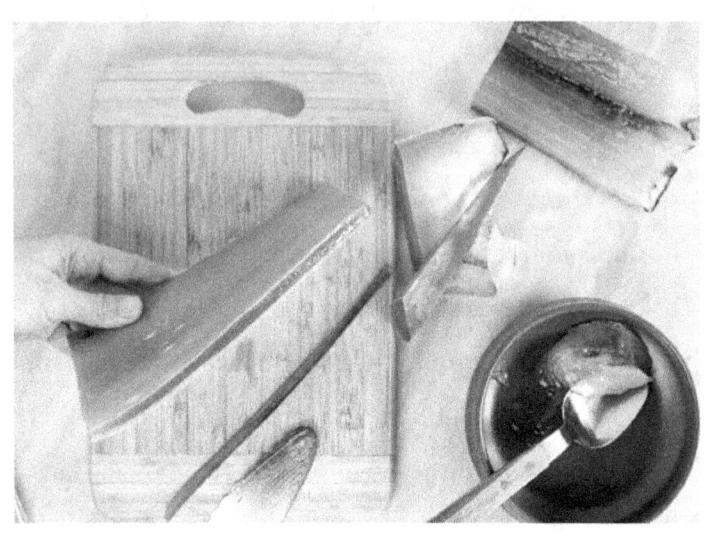
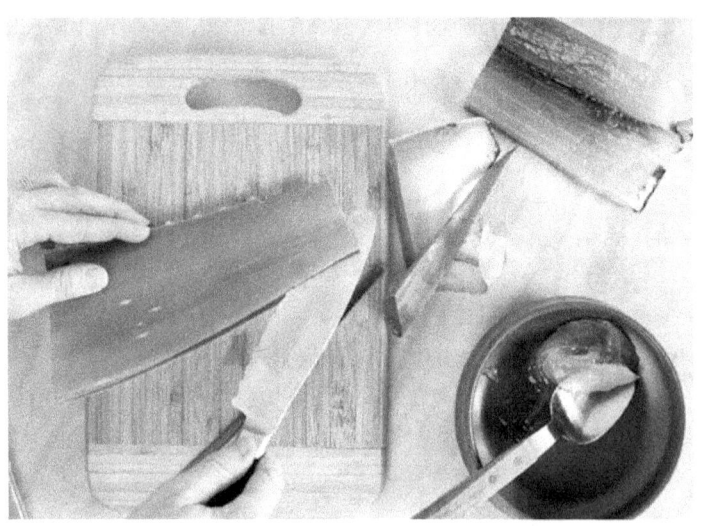

The best approach is to only use a spoon to scrap the green content off the Aloe Vera gel.

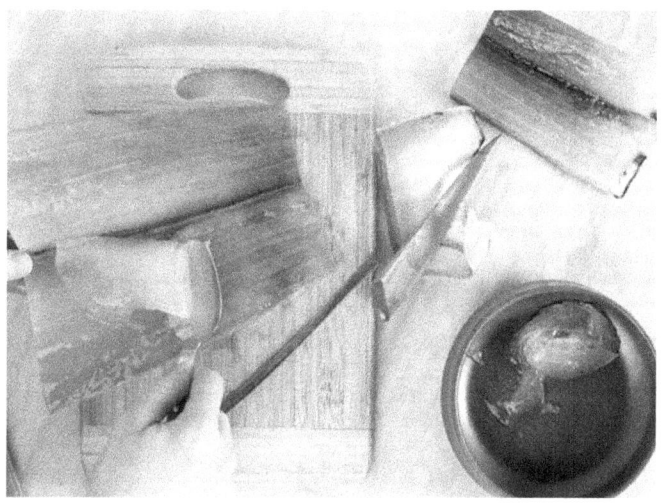

Place the aloe in a saucepan and wash off any yellow sap under cold water. For this recipe we will just require 1/4 cup Aloe Vera gel, you can easily weigh the part to mix and then preserve the remainder of the aloe in chunks to transfer to the smoothies or save for summers sunburns!

A reminder about frozen aloe, the consistency varies from frozen after the thawing. The gel becomes less rigid and waterier, it's barely noticeable in smoothies but it has a lighter, more watery quality for topical skin procedures.

Steps

HOW TO MAKE FRESH ALOE VERA HAND SANITIZER

To produce this fresh Aloe Vera hand sanitizer, we should mix the aloe to split it down entirely, then mix it with alcohol once again. For this method you can use a mixer, food processor, or bullet style blender.

Isopropyl alcohol is the ideal disinfectant to be used to make a hand sanitizer with homemade Aloe Vera- it has an alcohol concentration of ninety-one per cent. Secondly, a highly tested grain alcohol like Everclear- will be seventy five percent -ninety five percent alcohol. Because most cities and grocery stores are presently out of the above products, you should use high-proof vodka (or other alcohol) as an alternative, ideally with alcohol of sixty five percent -seventy-five per cent.

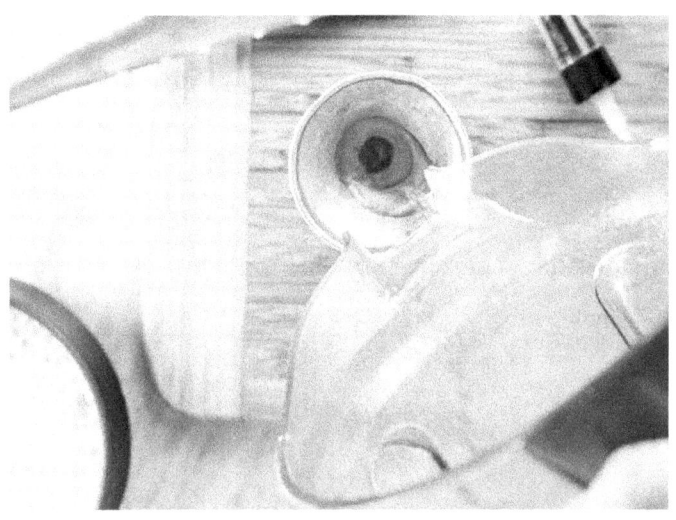

Here's the skinny: Hand sanitizer requires at least sixty percent of alcohol to be approved by the CDC to be safe. A sixty per cent alcohol, calls for high-proof vodka, right? True- when we dilute the vodka with Aloe Vera gel, this sanitizer is going to drop below sixty per cent. Using a fifty percent vodka with alcohol may further reduce the amount of alcohol. Make logical sense?

What should you do? This recipe is aimed to assist those people who have no significant exposure to hand sanitizer, isopropyl alcohol, or Everclear. Most shops in our city do sell Aloe Vera gel.

DIY SANITIZER ALCOHOL PERCENTAGES

The given table is an approximation focused on the alcohol evidence used for the ultimate percentage of this hand sanitizer formulation. This is only an estimate, which can't be assured.

Base Alcohol %	Fresh Aloe Vera	Alcohol	Final Estimated Alcohol %
80 proof 40%	1/4 cup	3/4 c	30%
100 proof 50%	1/4 cup	3/4 cup	38%
120 proof 60%	1/4 cup	3/4 c	45%
151 proof 75%	1/4 cup	3/4 cup	56%
Isopropyl Alcohol 91%	1/4 cup	3/4 c	60%
190 proof 95%	1/4 cup	3/4 cup	64%

CDC RECOMMENDED ALCOHOL PERCENTAGE

To order to safely remove germs and bacteria, the CDC suggests hand sanitizers be at least sixty per cent alcohol. Does a sub-60 per cent manual sanitizer harm germs, bacteria, and viruses? While this mix might not be as powerful as a sixty per cent hand sanitizer, it also has a high alcohol content. That combined with the mechanical method of rubbing hands together through 20-30 seconds after application can also assist in removing microorganisms.

This DIY Aloe Vera hand sanitizer wasn't evaluated in the laboratory, I'm not a physician and I can't give medical advice. This is beyond range for the median household to evaluate the alcoholic content of the homemade hand sanitizer. (What do we say about the lack of research now?) Use this at your own choice.

Remember also: Improper use of hand sanitizers or handmade hand sanitizers that may have a concentration of alcohol greater than the average sixty percent, can have a rubbing impact on your hand. This can directly benefit, microscopic cuts and/or bruises on your hands possibly providing a microorganism point of entry.

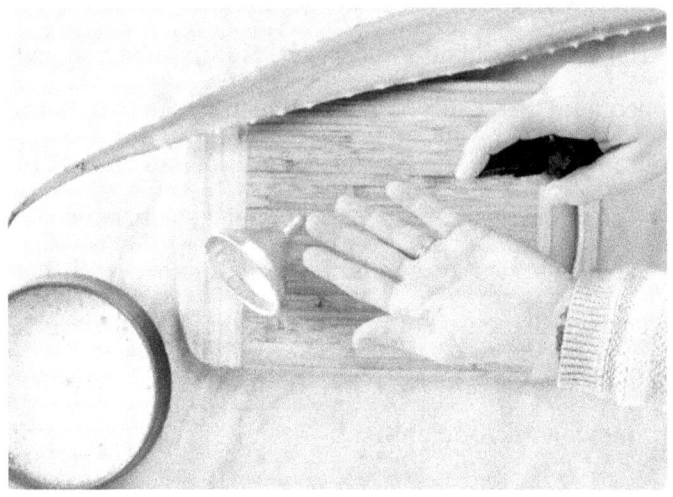

Hand washing is preferred overusing hand sanitizer!

Washing your hands for 20-30 seconds with soap and hot water is an efficient way to reduce the number of pathogens existing in our hands. We still do have handwashing, with or without a hand sanitizer, as an alternative to hold pathogens at bay!

Take priority of hand washing during hand sanitizer use, and make sure to moisten the hands after using hand sanitizer daily.

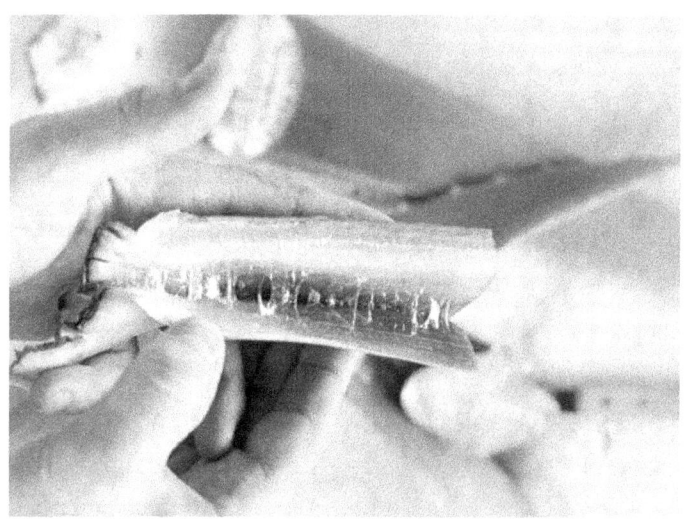

BENEFITS OF FRESH ALOE VERA GEL

Using fresh Aloe vera to produce your own Aloe Vera gel will make sure you get the decent things! When used medicinally on the skin, fresh aloe is admired for its hydrating moisturizer, cooling, and soothing effects.

That is included in the recipes of DIY hand sanitizer as its moisturizer qualities can help counter the drying that can impact high intensity alcohol on the hands.

Reading beyond the glossy front-facing logos and researching the panel of components to figure out the facts of what's really in a material is a custom that, sadly, we 're now getting more used to. Aloe Vera gel sold in supermarkets is another excellent example- most Aloe Vera product offered in shop shelves today contain various refined, organic, and preservative additives, with a relatively small percentage of real Aloe Vera for certain brands.

FRESH ALOE VERA + VODKA HAND SANITIZER

For DIY hand sanitizer recipes, fresh Aloe Vera and vodka can be a substitute when supermarkets are out of all traditional ingredients. This recipe gives you the choices to find your own hand sanitizer using away from the traditional recipes!

INGREDIENTS

- 3/4 cup grain alcohol
- 1/4 cup fresh Aloe Vera gel
- spray bottle

INSTRUCTIONS

1. Cut the Aloe Vera leaf at the root, the white part will diminish, and the leaf will be

green. Generally, 2″-3″ come from the leaf base.

2. Simply cut the upper portion skinny once narrowing to about 1″ wide.

3. Cut the aloe leaf's spiny surface down the side of one side to expose the freshly gel within.

4. Place your blade carefully between the Aloe Vera gel and the green skin as you filet a steak, holding your blade close to the green skin. Put the knife just below the green skin before you approach the other side of the blade.

5. Drop the knife, then pull the green skin softly off. Begin to slice and peel until completely exposed on one side of the aloe. Using a teaspoon to clean all the new Aloe Vera gel out and put it in a mixer.

6. Stand mixer for 15-30 seconds, before there are no foamy bits left.

7. Measure 1/4 cup of the Aloe Vera gel and the equivalent amount of isopropyl alcohol or grain alcohol after the label table. Merge the

unique blend once again for 15 seconds to complete.

8. Load into a bottle of water, and stock for up to 3 weeks.

9. Spray on your palms for 20-30 seconds and rub palms together.

NOTES

The ultimate percentage of alcohol can drop below the CDC prescribed sixty per cent alcohol solution for hand sanitizer, relying on the grain alcohol utilized.

So much use of a hand sanitizer may have a negative impact on the hands. Wash your hands for 20-30 seconds with hot water and soap where feasible.

Method 1: DIY Disinfecting Wipes (Natural & Reusable)

These DIY disinfecting wipes make it easy to keep your home clean without problematic chemicals. They're easy to make, natural, and reusable — just wash and reuse! Our homemade cleaning wipes are made without vinegar, so they're safe for use even on porous surfaces like marble & granite. Read on to learn how to make your own disinfecting wipes with essential oils.

While store-bought disinfecting wipes can be helpful for instant cleaning, they certainly aren't environmentally friendly or effective for your breathing.

Making DIY disinfecting wipes with non-toxic additives such as vodka, castile soap and antimicrobial essential oils is healthier for gentle clean-ups.

Number of studies have reported that specific household cleaning items can in fact cause asthma or other respiratory disorders in otherwise healthy people, especially supermarket-brand sanitizing wipes.

In addition, the pollutants from several store-bought household cleaners may trigger an assault in those who already have respiratory conditions.

Undisclosed ingredients in commercial disinfecting wipes

To add to the ambiguity, producers are permitted to retain customers in the dark on what precisely is in their cleansing products. Sadly, existing rules do not allow the listing of ingredient details on the product's packaging.

More and more cleaning product firms have suddenly started offering some product information on their business advertise. Though, those descriptions are also not accurate.

The Environmental Working Group site is a go-to for manufacturing companies are permitted to leave off their labels of the ingredient lists. The EWG also offers additional information to consumers — including the adverse effects and the rapid degradation of each ingredient.

Here's a comprehensive list of other famous brands and their products for commercial wash.

Even so, if learning about the harmful chemicals in cleaning supplies turned out to be fearmongering, or if you say, "but how can these handmade wipes disinfect my counter? "Well, tests have shown that the antibacterial, anti-fungal and antiviral properties of certain essential oils.

Top antibacterial essential oils for homemade cleaning wipes

Without all the bad side effects of store-bought cleaning products, the preceding essential oils (in no specified sequence) combat bacteria and household odors. This is worth remembering that essential oils are simply an addendum to the alcohol's sanitizing properties.

As long as the wipes formula also includes powerful disinfectants such as high-proof vodka (or rubbing alcohol), you can make disinfecting wipes with natural oils. Do not depend on essential oils as your primary disinfectant, particularly just after an effective epidemic of the virus.

Subsequently, you can replace any other mixture of antibacterial essential oils from this list with the essential oils used in the description below:

Essential Oils:

- Eucalyptus
- Lemongrass
- Tea Tree Oil
- Grapefruit
- Palmarosa
- Cinnamon
- Rosemary
- Bergamot
- Orange
- Clove
- Oregano
- Thyme
- Basil
- Lavender
- Peppermint

Unexpectedly, various studies have already shown that cinnamon is indeed the top performing important antibacterial oil.

Ingredients for DIY disinfecting wipes

In my homemade disinfecting wipes, I still use high-proof vodka which is a much more effective disinfectant. Vodka also serves as a non-toxic preservative that stops the fungus and microbes from developing. The alcohol level of the vodka brand you're using for this recipe is very relevant, however.

The brand should be at least Seventy per cent alcohol, since this is the minimum percentage necessary to kill a wide variety of bacteria and viruses while sanitation. That comprises such bacteria as E. Coli and lipophilic viruses, for instance influenza.

Vodka brands which follow the high alcohol level requirements usually involve:

- Everclear – 95% alcohol or 190 proof
- Spirytus Rektyfikowany – 96% alcohol or 192 proof

- Devil Springs Vodka - 80% alcohol or 160 proof

- Good ol' Sailor Vodka - 85% vodka or 175 proof

- Balkan 176 - 88% alcohol or 176 proof

- Pincer Vodka - 88% alcohol or 176 proof

When needed, the vodka can be supplemented with isopropyl alcohol (or rubbing alcohol) in this recipe. Important to remember, though, that isopropyl alcohol is highly inflammable, easily absorbed through the skin, and in some individuals its fumes can trigger blurry vision and migraine headaches.

Isopropyl or rubbing alcohol is also extremely poisonous if drunk, whereas vodka (or ethyl alcohol) is suitable for human consumption. Not like you're going to be drinking the wipe blend, so it's easier to use alcohol if you're trying to clean out places where little mouths are trying to be.

I recently saw DIY wipes vinegar and castile soap ideas but combining vinegar with castile soap can cause the mixture to coagulate. The acidic vinegar and alkaline soap would also nullify each other leaving their washing capabilities worthless.

Consequently, vinegar is not suitable for stone countertops. So, if you have stone countertops, be careful of any vinegar-containing DIY sanitizing wipes recettes. That said, vinegar is already a good natural disinfect for several domestic items and is healthy.

Save money on cleaning wipes with reusable cloths

You can even save money by making these DIY sanitizing wipes because it is easy to wash the t-shirt squares (or cloths) used in this remedy and then substitute them in a corresponding batch. That also ensures these wipes are consistent with an environmentally sustainable, low-waste lifestyle.

you don't have any old t-shirts on hand or want a thicker fabric, relying on your choice there are still several types of sustainable cloths accessible. Heavy-duty microfiber fabrics, cotton towels and biodegradable bamboo cloths are only a handful of the available options.

How to use these sanitizing wipes

Before using your wipes, involve a combination of soap and warm water to carefully remove and scrub the area of any dust particles, grease, or sludge. Any soil or contaminants left on your surface can impair your wipes' sanitizing capability, and this is a big measure.

These wipes can be stored in your bathroom and kitchen cupboard for easy, light sweep up of germ-prone domestic surfaces. If ease is a plus for you, you could also use these DIY disinfecting wipes on the go, and you can convince them to be independent of brutal antimicrobial agents such as triclosan.

These wipes are also secure enough to be used on palms but make careful to use specific skin-safer oils such as peppermint, lavender, tea tree, and eucalyptus, and do not reach the mouth or skin upon use.

Even though, this should be mentioned that it is beneficial to wash your hands with soap and hot water. Even so, when you're not around a drain, those wipes are good than doing nothing.

DISCLAIMER:

Such cleansing wipes have not been checked in the laboratory to assess their efficacy towards viruses so kindly do not use them to this end. Each material used to cure viruses must have alcohol level of at least seventy per cent as required by the CDC as well as other medical associations.

Steps

DIY Disinfecting Wipes (Natural & Reusable)

Such handmade wipes wash and disinfect, without toxins, hands, and kitchen floors. Rather than brutal antimicrobial agents, made with vodka, castile soap and essential oils. No alcohol with an isopropyl! Environmentally friendly, recyclable, and non - irritating

What You'll Need

INGREDIENTS

- 1 cup high proof vodka
- 2 1/2 - 3 tablespoons castile soap
- 20 drops lemongrass essential oil

- 10 drops tea tree essential oil
- 10 drops eucalyptus essential oil

SUPPLIES

- Mason jar with cover or a disinfected container
- Old white t-shirt trimmed into pieces (or microfibers or other simple cotton towels)
- Sticky water-resistant label

INSTRUCTIONS

1. Squeeze the vodka into your mason jar.

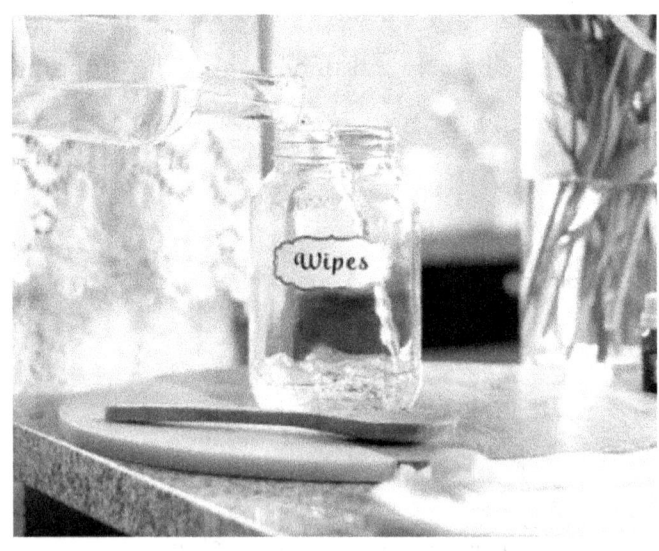

2. Introduce the essential oils that will quickly mix with the alcohol. Stir to mix strongly.

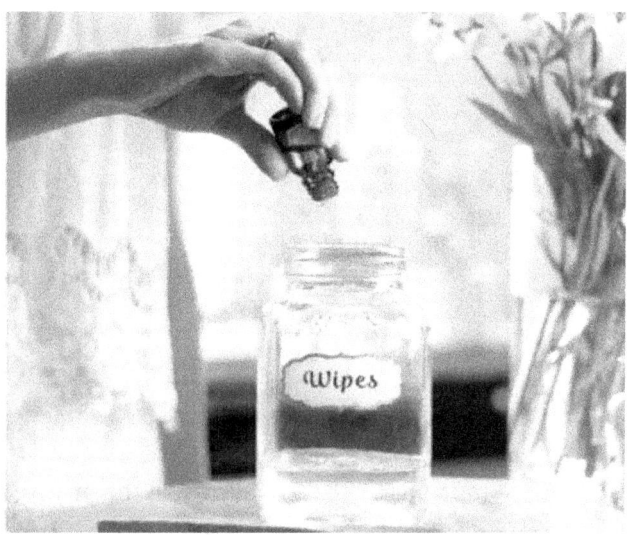

3. Introduce the soap, then wiggle it softly into the mixture. Make sure that trembling causes the castile soap to sudden.

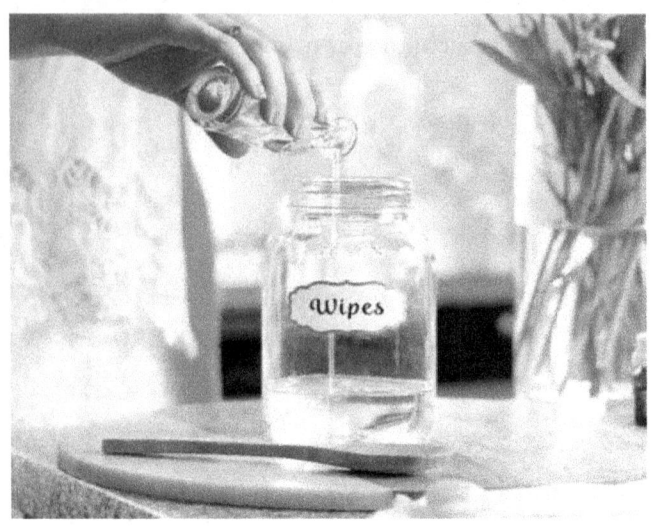

4. Wrap your cloths as is shown in the picture and put them in the container of the mason.

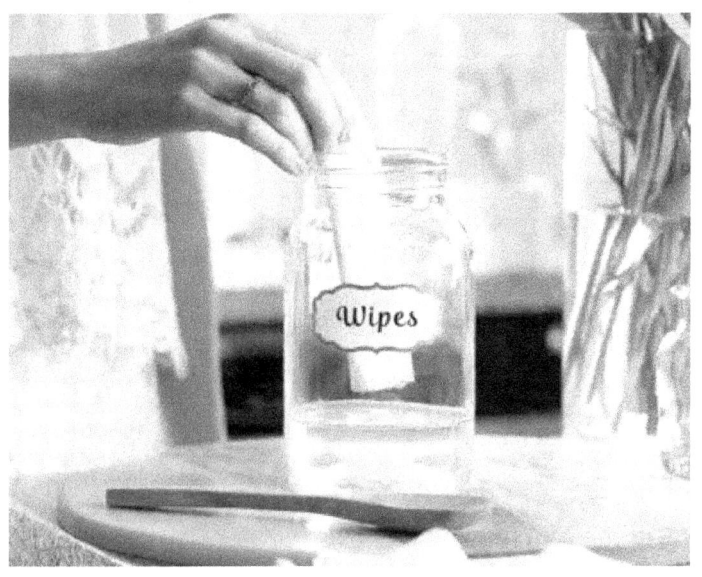

5. Replace the cap and gently swirl again so that the cloths get drenched with the solvent.

6. Keep the disinfecting wipes in a cool, dark spot, like under the kitchen or bathroom tap, with the cover securely closed.

Notes

If stored properly your DIY disinfecting wipes should last about 3-4 weeks. We don't advocate keeping items in plastic bottles or cans with large levels of essential oils. From all our DIY goods, we use glass storage boxes for essential oils, since essential oils are highly active and can leach contaminants from plastic containers. Please review your healthcare professional regarding the use of essential oils, particularly if you are pregnant or breastfeeding, have allergic reactions or have tiny kids in your residence. Other essential oils such as rosemary, clove, and eucalyptus to be used during breastfeeding are opposed. It is also important to avoid other essential oils such as rosemary, peppermint, oregano, and eucalyptus, or to use them with precaution with kids below 10.

Method 2: DIY Sanitizer Wipes at Home

Over the pandemic, sanitizing wipes became highly impossible to locate on the store shelf, but we need them more than ever to prevent getting infected. If shops are out of Clorox Wipes or Lysol Wipes near you, you can make your own disinfectant wipes at home, but you have to use the right recipes to make them efficient. The CDC has clear disinfectant protocols, and, in the pandemic situation, they are highly worth noting.

What ingredients work for disinfectant wipes?

Indeed, there are quite few other hygiene items that you can use to combat against virus in sanitizing wipes. Did not make it to shop or were online stores cleaned from what you want and need? This is how to get the most out of what you've got in your home.

Alcohol

You need at least seventy percent alcohol and in fact, that much 80-proof vodka is just 40 percent alcohol.

Utilize booze that is at least 140-proof, such as Ever clear, Golden Grain or Spirytus Vodka, if you were to definitely raid your liquor cabinet for antiseptic reasons. Domestic rubbing alcohol is successful as long as it has an alcohol content of at least seventy percent.

Hydrogen Peroxide

Hydrogen peroxide can be used as a sanitizer as long as it is 3 percent — but retain it in a black or dark bottle, as the chemicals are unstable when get interaction to light.

Bleach, Lysol, Pine-Sol, and other antiseptic cleaning products primarily marked.

Using bleach or Pine-Sol, and items of the Lysol type — be very sure that the container says it is a true antiseptic, because not all of these goods and their numerous varieties have sanitizing properties. Like bleach these items can be combined with water and dissolved. The best approach here is the ratio: You need five teaspoons (or 1/3 cup) of bleach per gallon of water, or four teaspoons of bleach per quarter of water for small volumes. Like other items, their tags provide a reference to the water-to-product antiseptic ratios.

What doesn't work for disinfectant wipes?

Use ingredients such as essential oils and other forms of "holistic" cleaner because they do not actively kill germs or pathogens. The white vinegar, vodka and lemon juice don't work anymore. If you want to add essential oils for scent, that's acceptable — just make absolutely sure you 're not depending on them in your product as the real disinfectant.

How can I make disinfectant wipes with bleach?

Here are the following steps:

- Hold and cut a roll of structurally sound paper towels in half (a bread knife tends to work very well for that).

- Blend with two cups of water at a spoonful of bleach.

- Place any pair of your paper towels in an airtight bag.

- Put one cup of bleach solution into each tub over each of the rolls, then secure it.

How can I make disinfectant wipes without bleach?

If you are using Lysol, alcohol, or some other disinfectant rather than bleach, just adopt the disinfectant dilution ratio guidelines for the solution given by their bottle. When using hydrogen peroxide, make sure that those bottles are used in which the wipes safely are in dark and opaque.

What surfaces in my home are safe to clean with disinfectant wipes?

You want to make sure that the solution you use with your wipes and disinfectants is suitable for the surfaces that you will be washing. Review your labels and be sure it will not hurt, strip, or smear your products, for bleach or other disinfectant cleaners. Usually, disinfectant wipes are best suited to most hard, nonporous surfaces. These usually include the below but can vary your own house and its equipment:

- Countertops

- Trash cans
- Doorknobs
- Faucets and faucet handles
- Cabinet handles and knobs
- Drawer handles and knobs
- Toilets
- Light switches
- Remote controls
- Steering wheels
- Gear shifts
- Refrigerator handles
- Oven handles
- Microwave door handles

What else should I remember when using disinfectant wipes?

If you are using some form of disinfectant soap, make sure to be in a well-ventilated place. If bleach is used to make your disinfectant wipes, never use them with ammonia or any other toxin. Also be sure to give your disinfectant wipes sufficient time to properly kill the pathogen on surfaces — if you're not sure how long you need, verify out the directives for the EPA and CDC here.

Tips

How to Prevent From Virus

Either or not you are stocked up on the sanitizer, the CDC recommends that:

Wash your hands regularly: Nothing really beats washing your hands with soap and water for at least a few minutes. Hand sanitizer — including the actual, skilled stuff — should always be used while driving, even when you are unable to wash your hands.

Stay at home: But for important visits outside such as visits to the supermarket or to visit the doctor, don't leave the house. In location, that is also called sheltering.

Stay at least 6 feet away from other people: This is termed as distancing from society. Holding the gap makes it impossible for the virus to leap by respiratory droplets from somebody else to you (or vice-versa).

Wear a cloth face mask outside the house: The CDC now recommends everyone wear cloth face coverings when out in public where you may be near other people. Read out How to Make a CDC-Approved Cloth Face Mask (and Rules to Follow) guide to learn the benefit of a mask and how you should wear it. Kids under 2 years old should not wear a mask, nor should anyone who has difficulty breathing or taking it off. Do not buy or hoard medical-grade masks, like N95 masks. There is a massive shortage in the country, and the masks are needed by health care professionals.

Avoid touching your face: The virus can be transferred into your mouth from your hands.

Clean and disinfect frequently touched surfaces: Do it every day, particularly if you leave things or individuals, or enter your house.

Is It Safe to Use Vodka as Hand Sanitizer?

There are a number of different methods out there where individuals have used alcohol to manufacture their own home-made hand sanitizer, particularly because during the virus pandemic it is in high demand.

And, owing to the heavy demand, some distilleries also sell their alcohol to the hand sanitizer manufacturers.

So, while that might be accurate, you have to remember that in order to be fully successful, the hand sanitizer has to be at least seventy percent alcohol per amount, in that specific form. It's not always nice to just spill alcohol into your mouth.

There are vodkas out there that go up to ninety five percent alcohol, which will be successful, but much of the vodka you 're going to see is either twenty or thirty percent, which won't disinfect.

Homemade Facemask

Table of Contents

INTRODUCTION 67
ABOUT THIS GUIDE 69
PART 1: BASIC FUNDAMENTALS OF FACE MASK 71

    Why urge homemade fabric face masks now? 73
    What the CDC says about homemade face masks today? 74
    Some Mask Rules: 75
    Is it possible for everyone to wear a mask? 76

PART 2: TYPES OF MASKS 79

  SCIENTIFIC APPROACH TO MAKE YOUR OWN HOMEMADE MASK 80
    Choosing a material 82

PART 3: DIY YOUR MASK AT HOME 87

  NO-SEW OPTIONS IF YOU CANNOT SEW 87
    How to make a face mask with Grocery Bag 87
  HOW TO MAKE A NO-SEW FACE MASK WITH BANDANA, SCARF, OR HANDKERCHIEF 97
    Steps to Make It 97
    Alternatives to a Bandana, Scarf, or Handkerchief 101
    Alternatives to Rubber Bands 101
    Caring for Your Mask 102
  HOW TO MAKE A NO-SEW FACE MASK WITH A T-SHIRT . 103

PART 4: SEWN CLOTH FACE COVERING 107

  HOW TO MAKE A FACE MASK WITH COTTON FABRIC 107
    The right way to wear a face covering or cloth face mask 111
  APPROPRIATE USE OF NON-MEDICAL MASK OR FACE COVERING 111
    Non-medical face masks or face coverings should: 111

    Non-medical masks or face coverings should not: 112
    Can you reuse your face mask? 113

PART 5: CHILD SIZE FACE MASK 115

YOUR SUPPLIES 115
HOW TO GET KIDS TO WEAR A MASK 120
    Be Honest (But Not Scary) 121
    Get Your Kids Involved in the Design 121
    Turn the Mask into a Costume 122
    Make a Mask for a Buddy 122
    Do a Trial Run 122
    Offer a Reward 123
    Turn it Into a Game 124
    How to Use a Face Mask Safely 124
    Preparing to Wear the Mask 125
    Putting the Mask On 125
    Taking the Mask Off 126
    Keep in mind 127

PART 6: WHEN TO USE IT, WHY AND WHERE 129

WHEN TO WEAR A MASK AT HOME 129
    Whether you are wearing a face covering or not, the CDC still recommends that you: 130
    How to put a mask on and take one off 131
    Why masks matter more for this virus 131
    What precautions can I take when grocery shopping? ... 132
    What precautions can I take when unpacking my groceries? 134
    Homemade masks may help protect others from you ... 135
    Homemade masks may help protect you 137

LIMITATIONS 139

Introduction

A mask is not as good as the wearer and is not a substitution for physical distancing and proper hand hygiene. Everyone should have their own masks to use in public in a better environment to assist to prevent the infection from spreading secretly, and the CDC is currently considering suggesting that everybody use masks in public, not just people with indications.

Sadly, masks are a little difficult to get around right now, so purchasing masks limits the availability for health professionals who are in need of them. Even if the CDC does not issue a new guideline, it is possible that someone who cares about a suffering loved one will have at least a couple so they can sanitize one while carrying another.

Searching for the strategies to bring home your own face mask? If YES, then here is a full guide to continue with much less expenditures and no experience. When learning about face masks for VIRUS protection, there are usually three types: fabric homemade face mask, surgical mask, and respirator N95. Once you begin to make face masks, make sure you understand the difference between the styles, how they can assist to prevent VIRUS from spreading and the components you require. I understand you must have concerns, so I am breaking down what you have to learn about creating and wearing from hand-crafted masks to no-sew covers, and even bandanas tied to your ears through hair ties.

About This Guide

This guide is all about the **Homemade Face Mask** and it is unique from all of the others. The way the guideline is designed makes it easier to find the solution you are looking for. Go ahead and click the Guide to see for yourself. Nice bold headings direct your eyes to only the section you like, and you do not have to read the whole text for a quick response. This guide offers an exhaustive description of all facets of DIY your mask at home. Need details about how to get started? Here is the description too. So, place this tutorial up on your bookcase in a prominent spot. We are confident you will go back to that again and again.

Part 1: Basic Fundamentals of Face Mask

In its suggestion the CDC stresses the use of "face coverings," not simply "face masks." So, what is the distinction? Every fabric that protects the nose and lips, like a scarf or bandana wrapped across the forehead, may be a face mask. A face mask relates to a more particular design, which typically includes padding which is more suited to the nose, lips, and head, as if using ear bands.

Mask guidelines will quickly get confused, as not all masks are completely equal. Other than handmade caps, even medical practitioners, who are prone to the maximum VIRUS levels, are in severe scarcity. Sometimes, they are hard to match properly. The CDC does not suggest them for overall use, for these purposes. The CDC also does not suggest surgical masks to the public at large, due to a shortage. Such masks do not fit against the face but have nonwoven layers of polypropylene and are immune to moisture. Homemade cloth masks are the safest for general population.

Fabric masks which are officially approved by the CDC for common use. Fabric masks often let air in through the edges but neglect non-woven sheets that disperse moisture. They just hinder about 2 percent of ventilation in.

Except the other way around, what? When a mask holder coughs or snores, the membrane may be adequate to absorb a lot of the original nastiness jet — even if there are holes in the cloth or along the edges. The goal of the new mask experiments was to answer this: whether handmade fabric masks did a great job of virus confinement. Yet their downside is that DIY face masks are easily accessible and by chatting, coughing, spitting, and snoring can help alleviate the large particles that are expelled.

Why urge homemade fabric face masks now?

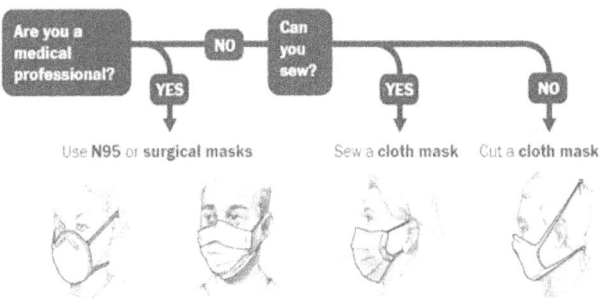

The CDC has suggested facial masks for months for those who were suspected to be or reported to be infected with VIRUS, as well as for emergency care staff. There are also evidence suggesting there might be some value of using a DIY mask of busy areas such as the store, as opposed to no face shield. Physical detachment and handwashing are also of utmost importance.

All persons wearing the masks may provide a level of membrane defense against respiratory droplets which are snorted or sneezed around them. Initial reports suggest that, after an infected person has left an environment, the virus will survive in particles in the air for up to one to three hours. Wrapping your skin helps keep any particles from hitting the air and contaminating others.

What the CDC says about homemade face masks today?

The most significant lesson from the CDC's warning is that it is a "voluntary global health initiative" to hide your face as you leave home and does not override established measures such as home self-quarantine, physical distancing, and extensive sanitizing.

In the terms of the CDC it "prescribes wearing cloth face covers in public places where other physical distancing steps (e.g. grocery stores and pharmacies) are difficult to maintain, particularly in areas with substantial community-based distribution.

CDC should not search for medical or surgical masks on its own and keep N95 respiratory masks to nurses and doctors, alternatively opting for fundamental clothing or fabric face masks that can be cleaned and recycled. The organization actually considered homemade face masks a last-ditch effort in clinics and hospitals.

Even a clear mask is very helpful in catching particles from your sneezes and cough. A recent survey has been reported to exhale into a giant tube, filled of multiple viral infections (influenza, rhinovirus, and a more moderate form of virus). Occasionally they didn't cover their noses and mouths; other hours they used a plain, not-particularly-fit mask.

The contaminated men, without the masks, exhaled infectious droplets and pollutants, small particles that lingered in the soil, about Thirty percent of the time they were examined. This covered almost Hundred per cent of virus particles but some of the aerosol particles while the sick people wore a mask.

Looking at all the findings together, we found that the bulk of virus-laden respiratory droplets and some virus-laden aerosols could be avoided.

Some Mask Rules:

Do not buy the surgical masks and keep them. Medical professionals are already facing a crippling supply shortage, and we should not use surgical masks that might be used for sick patients and health professionals.

Do not place a face mask on children under the age of 2—or anyone who has trouble breathing or may not be able to take away the mask themselves.

Do not cover a mask by the area of its lips. Seize it by the ties. Rinse your hands when you touch it.

Is it possible for everyone to wear a mask?

At the moment the World Health Organization (WHO) states that just two categories of people can wear face masks, those that are:

- Infected and showing signs
- administering for people who probably suspects to have this virus
- This says the healthcare staff will have surgical masks secured.

For the public at large, masks are not suggested, because:

- They may be affected by coughs and snores from other individuals, or when they are placed on or removed

- Regular hand laundering and social distances are much more productive. They might offer a false sense of security

Part 2: Types of masks

N95 respirator masks: These masks fit securely onto the face and have the best filtration capacity, trapping 95 per cent of 0.3 micron or bigger particles. An N95 mask prevents health care staff who comes into contact with large doses of the virus when treating and conducting numerous patient treatment services. That standard of security is not required for the majority of us, and these masks can only be used for medical care staff.

Medical masks: Such are still in demand and cannot be used by emergency staff. Often referred to as surgical masks or operation masks, these masks are square shaped garments which come with flexible ear loops. Medical masks are constructed from paper-like nonwoven stuff and are often offered to a patient waiting for a physician to see. Relative to the N95 mask, a medical mask removes between Sixty to Eighty percent of particles and also covers "large-particle droplets, splashes, sprays or splatters that may comprise pathogens," according to both the Food and Drug Administration.

Homemade fabric masks: The Centers for Disease Control and Protection advises that, when we are in public places, we shield our faces with a blanket or DIY cotton mask. Homemade masks differ in efficacy depends entirely on the cloth used, texture and design.

21 people have made their own masks out of T-shirts from another survey, and analysts compared the DIY masks to the surgical masks. "All masks considerably decreased the number of pathogens ejected by volunteers," the researchers wrote, even though the surgical masks were safer. Homemade masks have been found in group experiments to provide some security against viral infections.

Scientific approach to make your own homemade mask

Keep in mind that any facial covering is safer than no face cover. Although certain individuals use air filters and ventilation bags to play with DIY masks, the average individual does not require that degree of security if you exercise physical distancing and leave the house only for the crucial. Given that there is so much variety in materials, a light check is the safest recommendation. Keep the cloth or mask against the light, to see how much light falls. The stricter the weave, the less light you are going to see and the more preservation you get. However, check the cloth over your face to ensure that you can indeed breathe through this one.

Researchers have been studying everyday products because of a lack of masks to see how well they could fit in a handmade mask. They also related the volume and scale of the diluted molecules to the normal used by surgical masks — 0.3 microns. Checking two surfaces of materials use around 1-micron particles though. An analysis shows that the 0.3-micron check is an awesome quality, the 1-micron test will also be important to assist people to have a choice about mask substances.

"In 1-micron droplets / aerosols there are possibly a lot of further viruses than in 0.3-micron droplets / aerosols." "And even though a mask absorbs just 20 percent of 0.3-micron droplets / aerosols in thickness, it usually performs best with 1-micron droplets / aerosols, synthetic biology."

Here is a glance at some of the daily products that have been tested for homemade masks. You can check out so much in this book, What's the Right Material for Mask?

Choosing a material

T-shirts: Many of us have an old T-shirt which we could turn into a no-sew mask. It is one of the best common materials to use, but there is a great deal of variation in how well T-shirt clothing works in laboratory studies. A single sheet of an old cotton T-shirt caught twenty per cent down to 0.3 microns of molecules. It trapped Fifty per cent up to 1 micron of molecules. Two T-shirt sheets that trapped about Seventy per cent of molecules down to 1 micron.

Cotton quilting fabric: For its toughness this is the strong-thread-count synthetic fabric favored by quilters. Safety masks constructed from quilting cloth rivaled the filtration capacity of surgical masks in tests.

Tea towels: The tea towels are a common source of material for masks. Researchers have found that coating good in contrast to a 1-micron molecule scale medical mask. The creators of the analysis did not take care of the mark. The towel utilized was not a terry fabric, but a finely knit array of absorbent tea towels.

Pillowcases: Pillowcases are a great choice for sewers that have no other fabric. Two pieces of pillowcase fabric evaluated near to the effectiveness of the surgical mask at the 1-micron specification, but in a research, four layers of 600-thread-count pillowcase stuff were needed to attain the 0.3-micron conventional amount of security.

Flannel pajamas: One of the finest evaluated was a two-layer mask of flannel and silk which paralleled the reliability of a surgical mask.

Coffee filters and paper towels: For additional protection, the C.D.C. recommends putting a coffee filter into your mask. It is discovered that three coffee filters have made breathing difficult. Including a sheet of paper towel among two sheets of cloth will keep the handmade mask quite effective and a single paper towel filter twenty-three per cent of 0.3 microns and two paper towels filter thirty-three per cent. Our handmade T-shirt mask was applied with a paper towel.

Scarves and bandannas: You cannot top a mask or bandanna to shield your face when it comes to user kindness. Yet bandannas are small, that do not provide enough security, even rolled over four days. Scarves may be safer, but they can be warm and heavy. Both are safer than almost zero.

Optimally, the face mask of the bandana will blend snugly with your face and there are no spaces between your face and the mask. But you do need to make it easy, so you will not be able to change or re just the mask. If you should contact the front of the mask, washing your hands with sanitizer Lysol, or warm water.

Filters and vacuum bags: Researchers who are seeking to identify successful solutions for medical personnel have hacked down air filter layers and checked HEPA vacuum bags. Both can operate very well, but there are major disadvantages to both. When cutting air filters can unleash fibers that may be harmful to inhale, so if used in a mask the filter stuff should be wedged between layers of heavy cotton fabric. Vacuum bags are fine filters, but they are not so breathable. Besides, some vacuum bag brands can include fiberglass so do not use it to hide your face.

Part 3: DIY Your Mask At Home

No-sew options if you cannot sew

If when it comes to sewing you do not know where to start, there is a no-sew face mask choice. You should use tissue glue and an iron rather than stitching the cloth together. The iron is being used to weld together tissue and glue. You will also use the iron to make pleats for a stronger mask in the cloth.

When you do not have either of those items, you can use a scarf and some hair ties or elastic bands to create a face mask easily — once, this is for individual purposes.

How to make a face mask with Grocery Bag

Let us make this very clear: Masks are not assured to guard you from VIRUS, no matter how efficient.

This guide is an easy project for those with no sewing machine. Although cotton is requested in several ventures. There is no suggestion that it is better or bad than other textiles — it is cozier, and people want to keep it on hand. According to the theories of experts about the hydrophilic (water-loving) properties of the cotton masks that lead to increased levels of respiratory infection. Usage of a plastic hydrophobic substance identical (but not identical) to that used in surgical masks. And many individuals in their own home do get it right.

Tools

- Needle and thread
- Scissors
- Ruler
- Clothing iron
- Sewing or safety pins
- Permanent marker
- (Optional) Seam ripper

Materials

1. Medium non-woven polypropylene reusable grocery bag
2. Pipe cleaners (or plastic-coated twist ties)
3. (Optional) 60 inches of ribbon, between ½ and 1 inch wide

Instructions

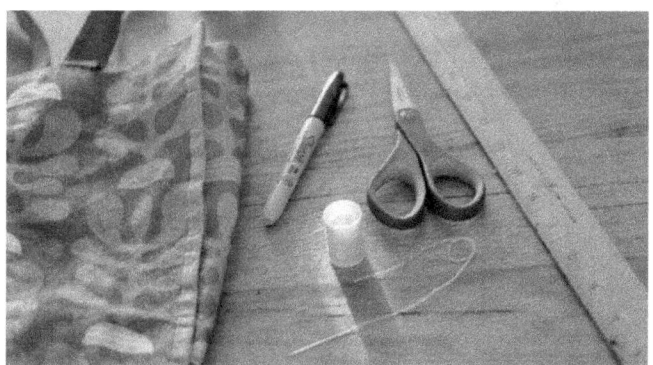

1. Wash the reusable grocery bag.

Caution: We explicitly suggest a reusable, non-woven polypropylene shopping bag (NWPP for short), not a reusable plastic one. It may sound stupid, but you have to breathe via the mask. Keep away from insulation packs (these normally have some inside foil material) or protective plastic lined containers, too.

Note: Pick the bag with the biggest handles you can get if you can. If you can use them as braces for the mask this design would be simpler. If the loops are not long sufficient, we will clarify how to construct ribbon belts.

2. Cut the sides off the grocery bag so the material lays flat. Do not cut off the handles.

3. Cut the material into two sheets. If your bag has a seam at the bottom, cut it like you did the side seams. You will get two clean sheets of NWPP, each with its own handle.

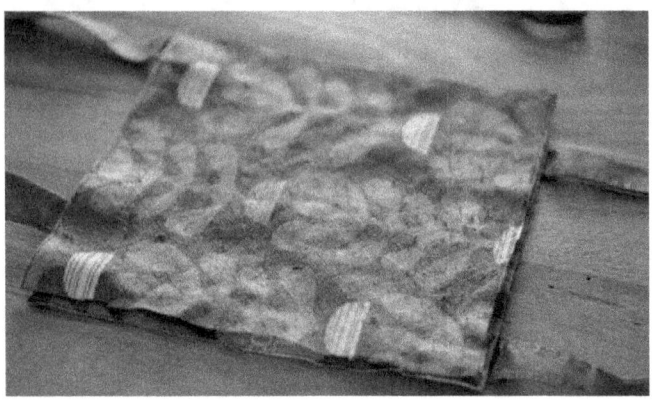

4. Measure and cut one sheet. Evaluate the top edge of the bag with the scale to reach the middle. Place your permanent marker on it. Using that as a point of reference, calculate back 4 1/2 inches and trace again against each stick. Calculate 9 inches from each point and make parallel vertical lines of cutting. Link the down lines. You must have a 9-by-9-inch square at the highest level with the clamp, with a completed (sewn) edge.

Note: When the handle is too big to fit within the square you have weighed, skipping over **(step 8)** and then use ribbon substitute **(step 9)** is the easiest option.

5. Repeat Step 4 on the other sheet of material.

6. Sew the mask's side seams. Put one layer on the wrong side (the former interior of the bag) and pull half an inch of content from the rim of the handle opposite. Iron the fold to put on low pressure. Sew it from the bottom then a quarter inch. Position the other layer on the right-hand side (the previous exterior of the bag) and fold it in half an inch like all the other layer, iron it and stitch it a quarter of an inch from the bottom.

Caution: Polypropylene is a plastic sort of thing. The use of an environment with high temperature will melt it, destroy your task and, most definitely, your iron. If there is no setting for "poly" then choose the smallest setting (usually silk) and every it marginally if the fold is not set.

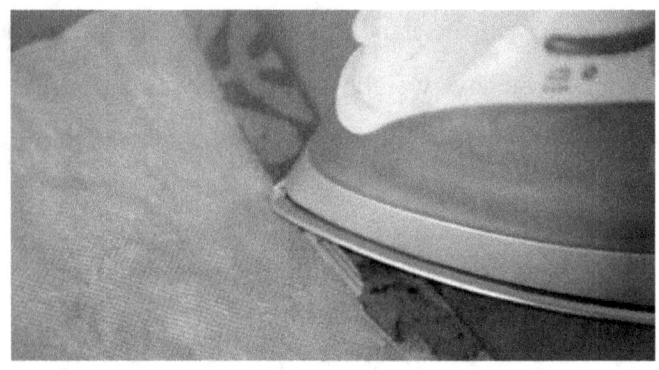

7. Place the sheets together. Your mask will have tissue on two layers. Position one of the layers on the work surface and approach the handle to the left. Position the other one over it, the handle confronting to the right. Pin on the spot.

Note: We suggest looking the same way on the illustrated side of the covers, because the back of the mask is a different color to the face. Davies claims this will better ensure that you do not misplace the mask, with the dirty side toward your mouth and nose, by mistake.

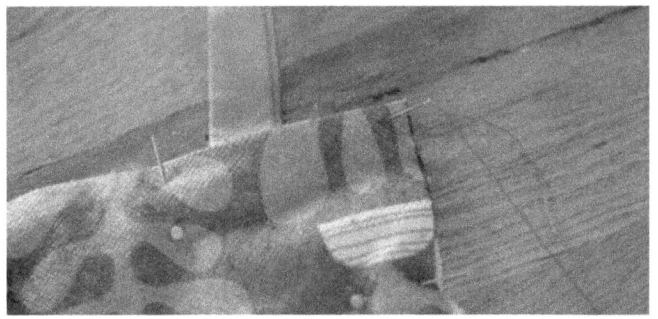

8. Make the head ties. Cover in half the handles and cut them in the middle. Keep the mask fixed over your face with loops sticking out from the bottom, and make sure the handles are long enough just to cover the back of your head with at least 4 inches to spare.

9. (Optional) Make straps out of ribbon. If your bag's handles are not long enough to even be belts, you'll have to build your own. Start taking the NWPP layers off the handles or use a seam ripper to clean them. Place the mask in the middle of your face and use the measuring tape to calculate the length of each brace — each brace should be sufficiently long to extend from the side of your neck to the back of your head and clip behind this one securely. Split the badges and pin them wherever the handles were. Placing your mask on check the fit. If the ribbon size is correct, dual your thread and sew the pieces on the wrong side of the sheets into place.

10. Sew the sheets together. Double your thread and sew all of the corners around.

11. Finish the bottom edge. Create a half-inch fold at the base as you did in Step 6, and iron it. Sew it shuttered from the rim by a quarter of an inch.

12. Make the adjustable noseband. Cover half an inch over the upper lip, then weld this again. Wrap or twist the pipe cleaners together and cut them to the exact width as the mask. Wrap in to break them at their ends. Inside fold tuck the metal bonds and pin the bend over them. Then stitch the fold underneath and on the sides of the links to secure them in position.

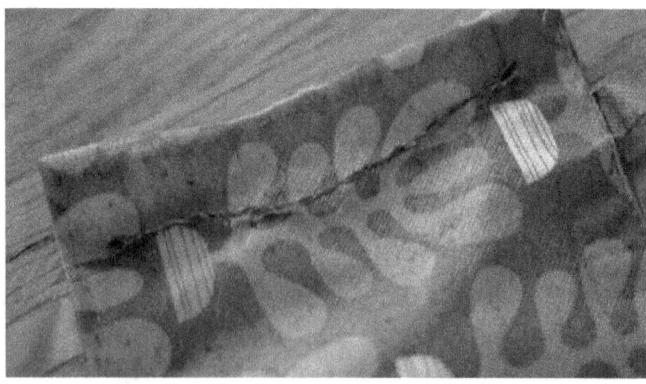

13. Make three folds to pleat the mask for expansion. Pleats should be about 1 1/2 "wide on the outside, half an inch broad on the inside, and overlapping to the nose band. If it benefits, trace the lines on the cloth, folded the rows and then iron them. Wrap this into place by sewing a quarter inch from the bottom of both ends. This time, twice the normal stitch back to ensure good plough edge.

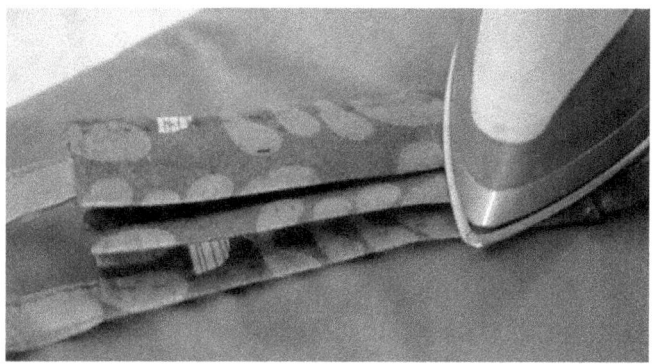

14. Sterilize your mask Immerse the mask in hot water for 10 minutes until first use. Undo the move between various uses.

Remembering one face mask simply is just not enough. Also make sure you bring glasses or sunglasses to shield your eyes and have never open the section covering your lips. Disinfect it when finished, let it dry thoroughly (in the sun if you have access) to avoid the bacteria from growing and then place the mask in a safe, waterproof, resealable container.

How to Make a No-Sew Face Mask with Bandana, Scarf, or Handkerchief

It is easier to make a no-sew face mask than you would imagine, which is a perfect option if you can't sew or don't have the right stuff. A no-sew mask is a fast task everyone can do — you don't have to be especially crafty or have needle and thread expertise. The biggest news is it takes just about five minutes to make it. Remember, you won't need to go out for materials, because this face mask guide just uses only things that you already have at home. At the end of this article we have mentioned possible tactical changes, just in case you don't have any of the recommended products.

Materials

- 1 Bandana, scarf, or handkerchief
- 2 Rubber bands

Steps to Make It

Only a few things you'll need to create your face mask no-sew. The bandana, scarf, or handkerchief has to be at least 20 inches by 20 inches, so covering your nose and mouth is massive enough.

1. Prepare Your Fabric

Use bandana, t-shirt, or other cloth that you want to use. Keep putting your cloth tight on the board, the shaped side experiencing the table and the back side confronting you.

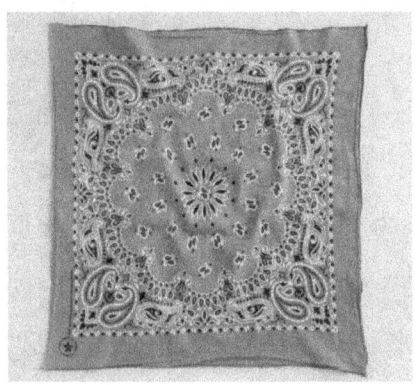

2. Make the First and Second Folds

Pick the top surface of the cloth and flip it over so that it meets the bandana center. Do that for the bottom half and folded up the cloth until it comes to the middle of the bandana, reaching the leading edge you folds down.

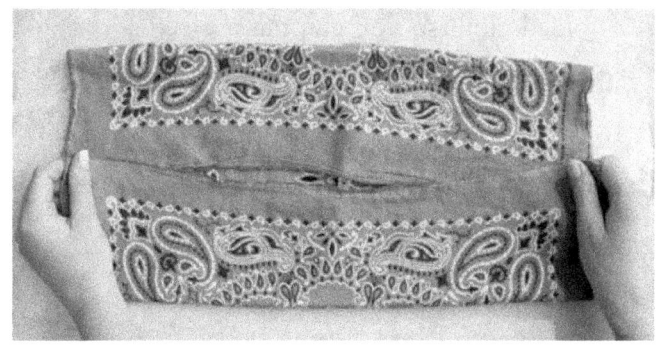

3. Repeat the Folds

Finish two further bulges by lining up at the top to the center and the underside to the middle. It will make a few pleats which will facilitate the mask to suit your face better.

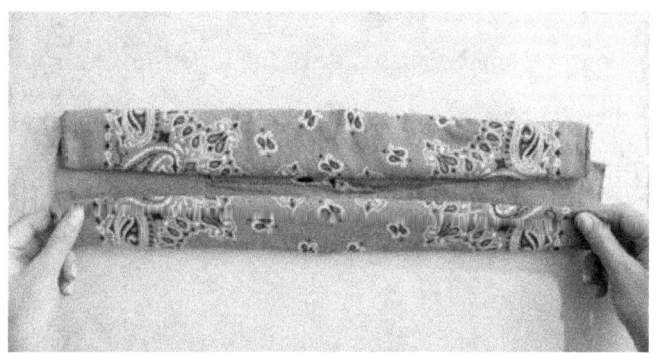

4. Fold the Ends of the Fabric

Wrap the right and left sides into the middle of the cloth rectangle. Now you'll have a shorter rectangle of folded cloth so you can put a piece of string on either side.

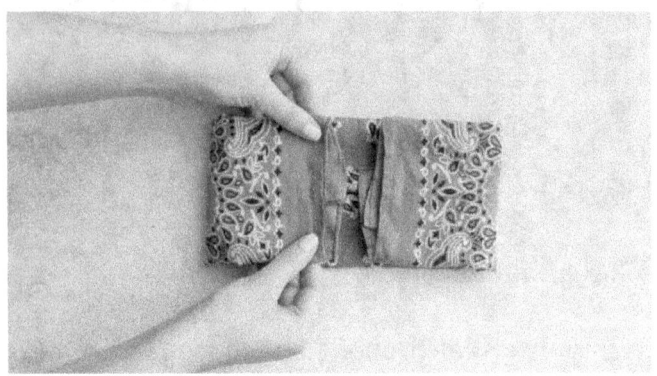

5. Slide on the Rubber Bands

Take a group of rubber and slide over one end of the rolled-up cloth, having left a few inches to the other. Continue on the other side of the rolled-up cloth, with the other rubber band. If you want you can curl one of those folds inside another to protect the fabric better, but that's not essential.

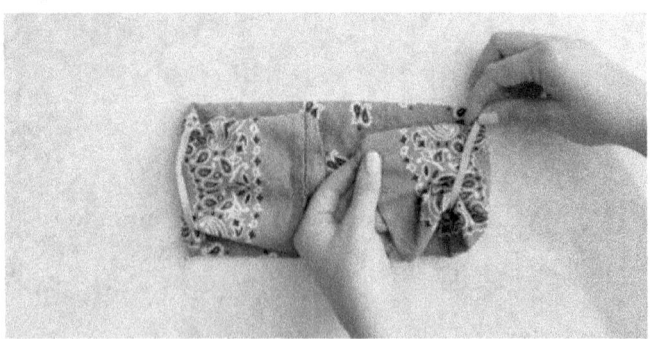

6. Finish Your No-Sew Face Mask

The side which faces you will be the mask's behind. Now, it's prepared to just use! Take the mask to your mouth to use and place the elastic bands around your ears to keep it secured. The mask would protect both lips and nose.

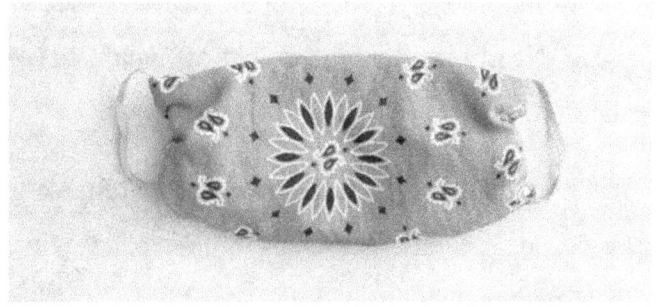

Alternatives to a Bandana, Scarf, or Handkerchief

You should cut an outdated piece of clothing if you don't have any of these things at. Textile cloth works likewise in a squeeze jersey garment from an old work. To make this no-sew mask, you will have to cut slits of fabric which is 20 "x 20."

Alternatives to Rubber Bands

If you don't have accessible rubber bands, there are a couple of other choices. When you have ties to the hair they're going to fit well. Only be sure they've got a lot of width on them.

There are several other choices if you don't have elastic bands or hair ties. You may trim an elastic loop from a set of pantyhose, tights, or leggings. You should take off part of the nylon cuff or the stretched part of the sole if you have an old pair of socks, just use it. Nearly any length you cut off would fit well about 1/2

Just note that whatever you are using to remove the hair bands has to be as stretchy as these bands will be the aspect that aligns over your head.

Caring for Your Mask

Such masks are wonderful for being usable and so easier to take care of. Only remove the elastic bands and clean the fabric just as you'd have a regular item of clothing. After every use it's suggested that you clean the cloth masks. To wrap your mask, keep reposting this tutorial, so you can dress up it once again.

How to Make a No-Sew Face Mask with a T-shirt

Steps

1. If you've got an old T-shirt, so you should transform it back into a face mask.

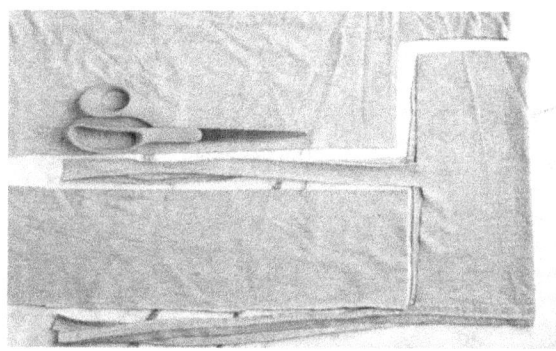

2. Cut this type out of a t-shirt beginning at a folded bottom. The two sections of rope should be about 12" long by 1" high, and the rectangle at the folding edge should be about 4" high by 14" large. When opened, the rectangle in the middle will be spanning 8" by 14".

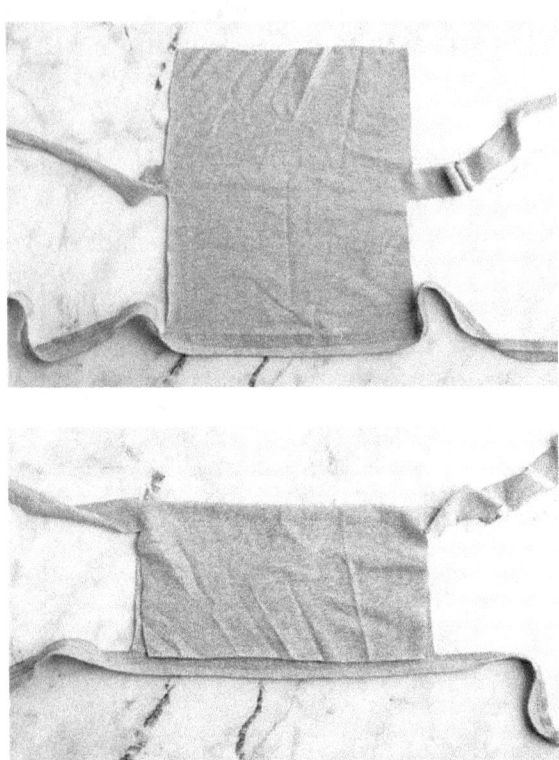

3. Place the slice of cut out and pull the top half down over the lower half. (That will show you two sheets of fabric on the main component of the mask.) After you've rendered that flip, there'll be four links at the four edges.

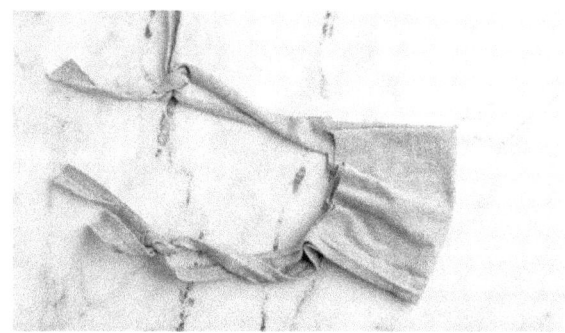

4. Knead the buckles behind head and behind the neck to dress up the mask. To change the fitting, you can put both braces behind the head

Part 4: Sewn Cloth Face Covering

How to make a face mask with Cotton Fabric

Materials

- Two 10"x6" rectangles of cotton fabric
- Two 6" pieces of elastic (or rubber bands, string, cloth strips, or hair ties)
- Needle and thread (or bobby pin)
- Scissors
- Sewing machine

Tutorial

1. Break out two 10-by-6-inch cotton print rectangles. Using closely knit cloth, such as cloth sheeting or quilting thread. T-shirt fabric is about to function in a small pot. Place the two rectangles; knit the mask as if it were just a single piece of fabric.

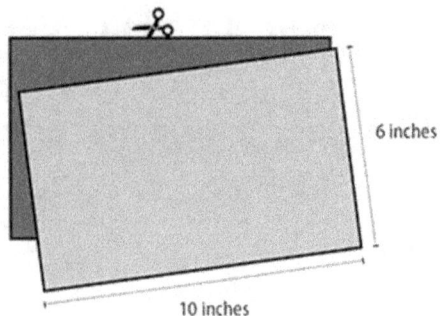

2. Fold in 1/4 inch and spread over most of the long sides. After which wrap over 1/2 inch over most of the short sides of the dual layer of cloth and sew down.

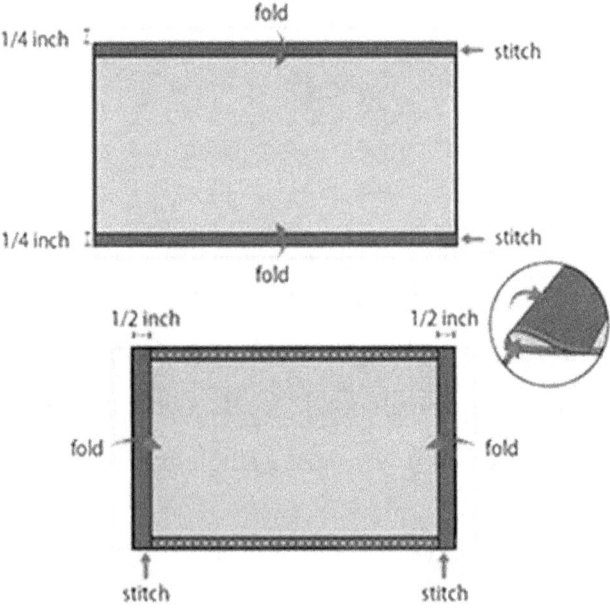

The top image shows the two bits of rectangular fabric which are piled on top of each other and meet on both directions. The triangle, standing straight, is placed so that the top and bottom of the triangle are the two ten-inch sides, while the left and right sides of the rectangle are the two six-inch sides. The top image shows the two long sides of the rectangle of fabric being folded over and sewn into place to create a one-fourth inch margin around the whole width of the rectangular top and bottom. The below image shows the two narrow sides of the rectangle of fabric being flipped over and stapled in order to create a one-half inch fringe over the whole range of the right and left side of the facial protection.

3. Pull a 1/8 "long rubber 6-inch length through to the wider fringe on either side of the mask. Those are going to be the ear cords. To loop it through using a wide needle or bobby pin. Bind the tight ends.

Aren't elastic? Using elastic head bands or hair chains. You can keep the links bigger if you just have rope, and bind the mask around your back.

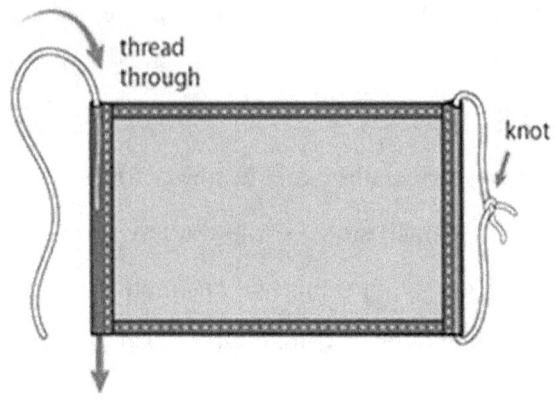

Two six-inch sections of rubber or rope are woven through the free, half-inch hems formed on the rectangle's left and right sides. Instead, the rope or string's two ends are bound together in such a band.

4. Push softly onto the rubber to tuck the loops within the hem. Pick the mask sides on the rubber and change the mask to suit the face. Instead tie the rubber tightly in order to prevent it sliding.

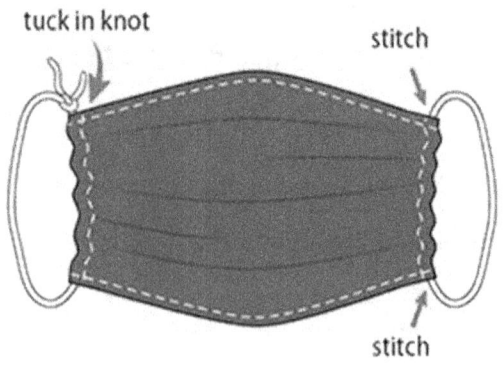

The right way to wear a face covering or cloth face mask

The first and most critical thing is to cover both of your nose and mouth, ensuring that the face mask will work under your jaw. When you're in a busy market, the shielding would be less comfortable if you take it from your face, like talking with someone. It is safer, for instance, to change your wrapping before you leave your house, instead of standing in line at the store. Check on why fit really is so critical.

Appropriate use of non-medical mask or face covering

An individual using a non-medical mask or face shield will decrease the spreading of his or her own contagious respiratory particles when properly attired.

Non-medical face masks or face coverings should:

1. Enable easy breathing
2. mesh safely to the head with ties or ear loops
3. to sustain their texture after washing and drying

4. to be altered as quickly as possible if humid or dirty

5. be comfortable and do not require regular modification

6. at least 2 layers of interwoven product fabric (such as cotton or linen)

7. be huge enough just to be completely and easily cover the nose and mouth

Some masks often have a pocket to hold a paper towel or coffee filter which can be disposed of for added advantage.

Non-medical masks or face coverings should not:

1. Be associated with other

2. compromised vision or conflict with activities

3. put on kids under the age of 2 years

4. composed of synthetic or other non-breathable materials

5. covered with adhesive or other unsafe items

6. made entirely of items that quickly break apart, such as tissues

7. put on someone unable to extract them without help or someone with difficulty breathing

Can you reuse your face mask?

Homemade masks and cotton fabric coatings are machine washable. Medical-grade masks are usually single-use but the extreme lack of N95 masks makes surgical limitations a must in many hospital conditions.

Part 5: CHILD SIZE FACE MASK

I set out to create mask model Child Size Face for you. This is really simple, and it takes only 10 minutes to do it, basically. For your and the children of your loved ones, you should make up a couple of these. This Face Mask for Child Size measures about 5"x 7". For various ages I'll send different measurements.

YOUR SUPPLIES

For ages 4-12- You require two strips of fabric measuring 5" x 7" and 2 pieces of 6" thick, 1/8th "rubber. If you are unable to obtain thin rubber, you should cut wider ones. Or if you can't seem to find some rubber, you should use long cords to attach them backwards.

For ages 2-4- You require two pieces of fabric measuring 4" x 6" and 2 pieces of 5" thick, 1/8th "elastic.

When your child has a large nose, you may choose to use rubber for further.

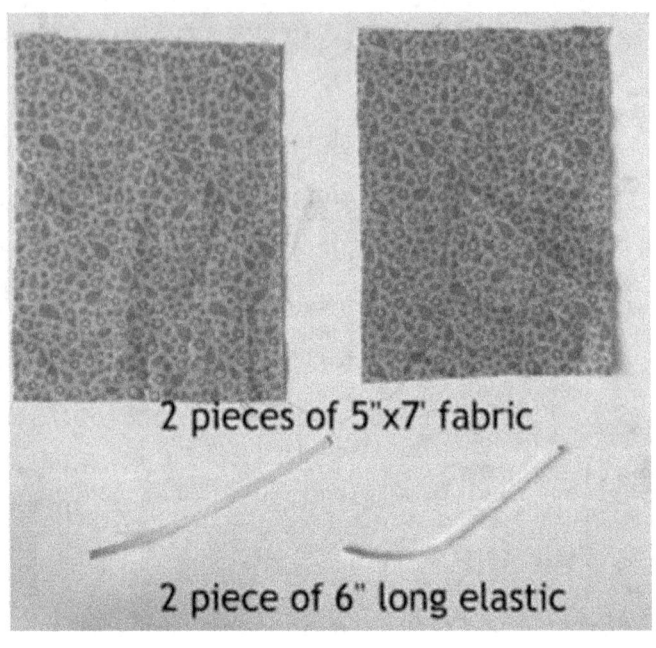

LET'S START SEWING

1. Pin elastic around 1/2" from small front side edges of a fabric.

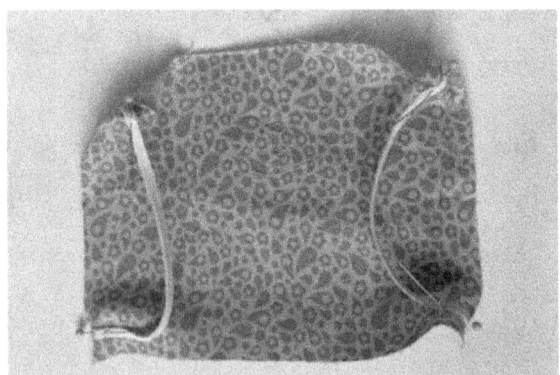

2. Then put the other piece of fabric face down on the right-hand side, and tie it all over.

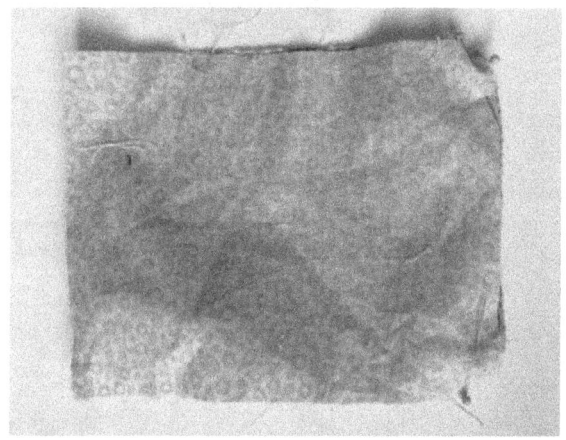

3. Sew the two parts of cloth all over linked. It can be difficult when you have the rubber corners so go slow. Left around 2" free, so that you can transform it inwards.

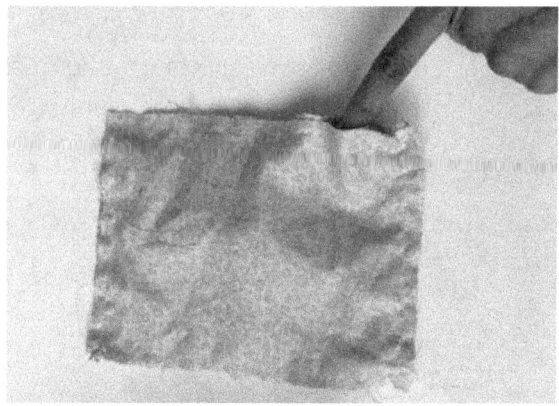

4. Turn inside. Wrap the gap down, then sealed the top sew.

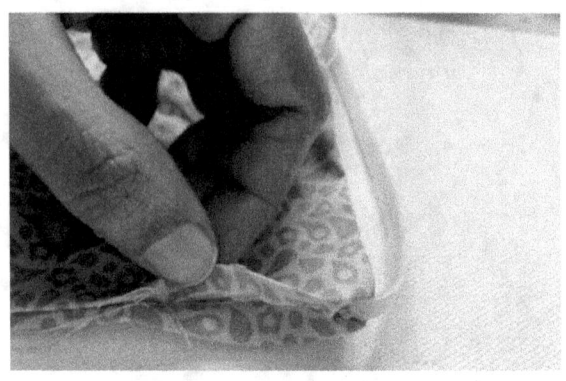

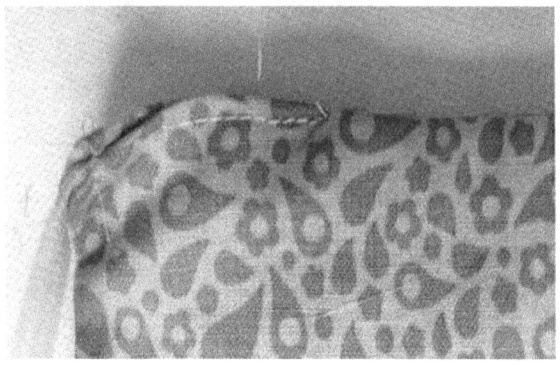

5. Then, do two sheets in the mask's side middle. The pleats are approximately 1" each.

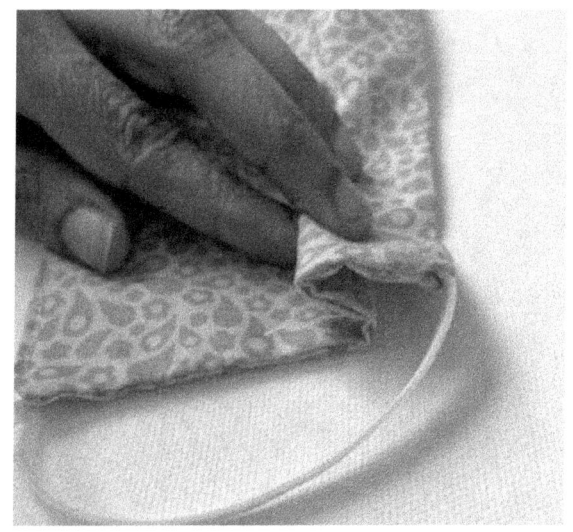

6. Place the folds and tie the ends.

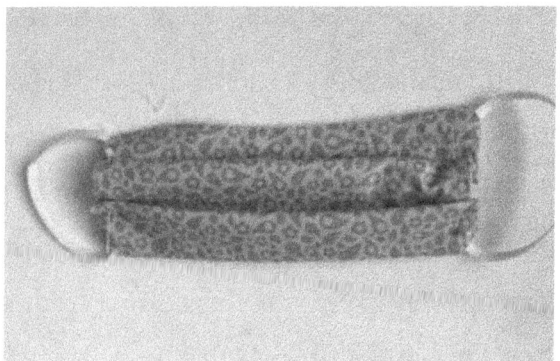

7. That is, it! You are done.

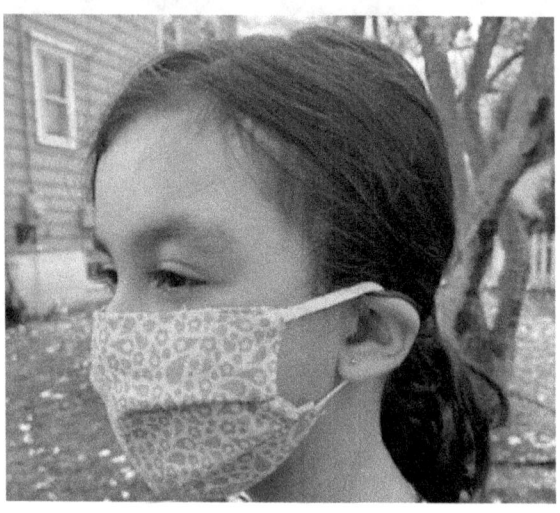

How to Get Kids to Wear a Mask

The safest choice in shelter-in-place and remain-at-home directives is to keep children at home with the other member of the family instead of taking them out. Overall, certain evidence suggests that children are not only likely to become carriers for the disease, they are also at danger of being sick. But when you really have no option but to bring your kids with you, you must have a mask on face.

Here are some suggestions to make the process go a little smoother

Be Honest (But Not Scary)

No matter how old your child is, be frank about why masks are necessary. You do not have to go into any details, and you should keep things age-appropriate so be transparent about the virus for your children.

Clarify to them that wearing a mask enables to protect the people around them. Avoid the temptation of dramatizing the circumstance or revealing more detail than is required. The idea of wearing a mask is then seen as an excuse to convey altruism and sympathy.

Get Your Kids Involved in the Design

One approach to get the children to buy into the notion of wearing a mask is to include them in the cycle of layout. Enable them to pick the pattern they want to use, such as an old T-shirt or a pillowcase featuring their beloved character in the cartoon. Just a simple white shirt or bed sheet they can put on can fit with textile paint. The trick to getting the fabric chosen for the mask.

Turn the Mask into a Costume

If you make a decision to use fabric paint on your kid's mask, assist them transform it into an animal or persona. To make a pup, small cat, or rabbit, it is simple, for example, to paint a mouth and whiskers on the mask. Mix that with some Halloween leftover eyes and you can notice your kids simply cannot wait to use their masks.

Make a Mask for a Buddy

Any kids may have a better risk of wearing a mask if their "buddy" wears one too. So, if your kid has an absolute favorite stuffed animal, an Old granny they're taking anywhere, or another beloved toy, make a mask for them too. And when you head out, they will come along with their partner as long as they have their mask too.

Do a Trial Run

For most kids wearing a mask is a unique experience. Yeah, the first couple of times the kids wear a mask, they can say it's itchy or they can't relax. Most kids aren't going to enjoy the thought of wearing a mask.

Check out the mask at home for this purpose. Let your kid wear it for 30 minutes. Exercise carefully putting it on and not removing it until it's mounted. Afterwards, explore how it feels to wear it for your family. And make modifications to the mask if necessary while also checking that it suits correctly.

Offer a Reward

Often children react favorably to what they're scared to do because they recognize there's a payoff at the end. As a consequence, you will inspire your children to wear their masks and give them something that will look forward to when they get home. For example, they might be receiving a badge for their poster, an ice cream cookie, or even an extra hour of TV to comply with the rules when out in public. You know what your child is inspired by so pick appropriately.

Turn it Into a Game

Other way to get your children inspired to wear a mask is to make it into a challenge. Creating a game out of wearing masks much like the "no talking challenge" or the "who can go the maximum without blinking" challenge. Have everybody start with 10 points, for example. They lose one point every time somebody moves their mask to change it. The one who has the most skill points wins game by the time you arrive home.

How to Use a Face Mask Safely

It's incredibly necessary to use a fabric mask properly. Otherwise you and your kids face the risk of potentially spreading diseases to yourself and others. In fact, the CDC advises that cotton face coverings will not be used for infants below two years of age. They can also not be used by someone who has difficulty breathing, is asleep or otherwise is incapacitated.

If your child is older than two years and relatively well, if you have to go out, it is usually appropriate for them to wear a mask. When you've cleaned the mask of your kid and it's prepared to go, here are few crucial measures to put the mask securely and successfully on:

Preparing to Wear the Mask

Clarify to your kids that it is time to start putting on their masks

Note that they could not contact the masks until they're on or removing them without permissions

Give sufficient time for conversation and attempt not to hurry your kid through the procedure, particularly if it's their first to wear a mask outside

Wash the kid's hands with soap or sanitizer before they contact the mask.

Putting the Mask On

- Pick up the mask by ties or clips with washed hands and properly attach it to your baby's face
- Making sure that the mask fits easily so that your baby still can breathe easily

- Change the cloth around the nose bridge to make it fit tightly (some people feel that holding your child's glasses or even sunglasses over the mask's edge lets her remain in place, but this is not needed).

- Be sure your kids are confident with their masks and warn them that they shouldn't contact it and leave it in place

- Clean your hand carefully, taking into account that you touched the mask and your baby's face

Taking the Mask Off

- Wash your hands until removing the mask and let your kid do the same.

- Note that the kids should not cover their face even though the mask has been taken away.

- Removing the mask through ties or belts

- Place the mask directly in the washer or in a plastic container.

- Wash the mask in a washing machine and make it dry in a drier.

Keep in mind

You should be washing your hands before and after each time you treat your face masks with your fabric. Furthermore, fabric face masks can never be used a second time before they are cleaned.

As well as being filthy from the saliva of your infant, the masks possibly contain pathogens and other pollutants. Keeping the mask on again without cleaning it just raises the risk of infection in your kid. In reality, a study published in the Lancet showed that the virus could live for at least one day on fabric and for up to seven days on surgical masks.

Part 6: When to use it, Why and Where

The suggestion is to wear a face mask in public places at all times, so we do not know who has the infection and who does not. Wearing a mask, particularly though you are indoors, is still more environmentally conscious. According to several authorities, outdoor activity, with or without a mask, remains relatively healthy. Research teams warned that little is known about heavy breathing and how it impacts viral proliferation during aerobic exercise. When someone tugs the mask off to reveal the nostrils. This can make the mask much less efficient when it comes to germ protection.

When to wear a mask at home

In the house, a mask is only required if somebody is sick. The patient should be limited to a single space with little or restricted interaction with the rest of the family (including pets) and can have, if feasible, a single toilet. All sufferer and caretaker will wear a mask when they came into contact.

Whether you are wearing a face covering or not, the CDC still recommends that you:

- **Wash your hands regularly.** Using soap and water for about 20 seconds, then wash them. If you cannot wash your hands, hand sanitizer is permissible to be used.

- **Hide your face** with a towel or the inside of your forearm while sneezing.

- **Stop touching your face**, since you can convey the virus in your throat from your hands.

- **Remain at home**, apart from important visits outside, such as visits to the supermarket or doctor's appointments. Of location, this is also called sheltering.

- **Experience distancing** physically by remaining at least 6 ft away from others. The White House also advises limiting 10 or more meetings which should be easy because you are sitting at home.

- **Wash and decontaminate regularly** hit surfaces daily.

How to put a mask on and take one off

- Clean your hands just first.

- Do not access the mask's cloth part — that is basically the germ barrier, so you do not want to disperse the germs it has captured.

- Use the ear knots or ties to protect and take away your mask. The coverage area will go down under your chin from above your nose bridge and extend to your ears around midway or more.

- Pull the links and loops so they align against your face as snugly as feasible. If there are pleats in your mask, the tucked side will be flat.

Why masks matter more for this virus

To begin with, it is a new virus which indicates that our immune systems have not had it before. It is different from the flu, from which many of us have some safety, either because of significant exposure to influenza-related viruses or because we have been shot. One of the greatest concerns is that there is no virus safety for health staff, who get screened to remain healthy through flu season.

It is also worth noting that the flu season occurs over many months. virus has spread much faster, infecting an abundant number of patients — and leading to tens of thousands of cases — in a matter of month.

An additional twenty five percent of virus patients feel completely normal and do not know whether they are sick and may be infectious. So, what are we to guess? You may well have been one of them! For this purpose, you must wear a mask to shield us from your concealed pathogens.

What precautions can I take when grocery shopping?

It is spread mainly by virus-containing granules, or through viral particles floating in the air. The virus can be effectively breathed in and can also distributed when a human hit a surface, or it is important to note that the flu season takes place over several months. virus has progressed even further, contaminating a large number of people — and resulting in hundreds of thousands of cases of — within a month.

An extra 25 percent of people with virus feel absolutely regular, and do not know that they are ill and may be contagious. And when are we to conjecture? You could have been one of them! To this end, you have to wear a mask to protect us from your secret microbes. An entity that carries the virus and then contacts your lips, face, or eyes. There is no existing evidence of a transmission of the virus by food.

Health measures enable you to prevent virus respiration or contact an infected area and contact your nose.

Keep at least 6 feet of space between yourself and other shopkeepers in the grocery store. Wash the frequently touched surfaces with hot water and soap such as grocery carts or basketball handles. End up having your face touched. Having to wear a cloth mask serves to warn you not to cover your skin which can also serve to prevent infection transmission.

Using hand sanitizer prior departure from store. Wash your hands the moment you return inside.

Restrict the visits to the grocery store if you are older than 65 or at higher risk for whatever cause. Ask a friend or roommate to pick up groceries and keep them outside your house. See whether your grocery store is offering special hours for older people or those with situations underlining them. Or have shipped supermarkets to your house.

What precautions can I take when unpacking my groceries?

Recent research has shown that the VIRUS could survive for up to 72 hours on materials or objects. This means that the virus on the surface of the grocery store should be denatured over the course of time after foodstuffs have been packed away. Try cleaning the outside areas or cleaning them with a sanitizer if you intend to use the goods within 72 hours. It will not infect the entire content of sealed bags.

Washing your hands with soap and water for at least 20 seconds, after unwrapping your groceries. Clean the surface areas you place on while unwrapping them with household cleaning products.

And that is when eating fruits and veggies thoroughly wash with water. And washing your hands before eating some meal you have taken home from the grocery store lately.

Homemade masks may help protect others from you

Homemade face masks cannot be able to eliminate any molecule and are not expected to protect you from contracting the virus, although under certain cases they may support. The extreme lack of N95 masks, which enables to deter the acquisition of virus by medical practitioners such as doctors and nurses, has indicated that ordinary citizens required a substitute to effectively stop the spread.

Using a fabric face mask while you're with people will help trap big particles that you could expel with a coughing, sneeze, or inadvertently released saliva (e.g., through speaking), which could delay the transfer to others if you don't realize you're ill. "These kinds of masks are not designed to protect the user but to prevent him from accidental exposure — in situation you are a virus symptomless carrier.

The only thing you can really do to keep virus from advancing is to clean your hands regularly for at least 20 seconds with warm water and soap. If none is accessible, using a hand sanitizer with an alcohol base of at least 60 per cent.

You can also perform the following parameters:

- Stay at home
- Keeping a 2-meter physical distance from others to shield you. If you cannot sustain physical space, try wearing a non-medical mask or a handmade face covering
- To prevent exposing your ears, lips, nose, or eyes

It has not been proved to shield the person who wears a handmade face covering / non-medical mask in the group and is not a replacement for physical distancing and washing hands. However, even though you have no signs, it could be an extra precaution taken to defend those around you. This would be helpful for brief periods of time where it is not possible to separate physically in urban spaces, such as when searching for food or using mass transport.

Homemade masks may help protect you

While we know that even a standard mask does a fairly better job of shielding the world from your outgoing pathogens, experts believe there's more variability in how well homemade masks could shield you from unspecified pathogens, based on the fit and reliability of the content used.

But the thing is, if you do practice physical distancing and cleaning your face, you do not need an extremely efficient mask. And if you use a cloth of good filtration capacity — like two layers of thick cotton or flannel — and wearing the mask appropriately, you are through the odds of virus avoidance.

The fact of the matter is that you reduce your risk of becoming sick when you start practicing physical distancing, washing your hands, and wearing a mask in those times when you just have to leave the apartment.

Limitations

Non-medical masks are not regarded as potent in obstructing tiny particles as the hard-to-get N95 respirator masks required by the medical profession.

All of this leakage in homemade fabric masks is why public health experts usually do not assume that wearing a mask hinders anyone from catching a virus which is already hovering around in the atmosphere. Flow of air takes the less resistant direction. When viral particles are in the area, they have an easy route around a cloth shield of their own making. And in the specific instance of a handmade cloth mask, people who wear might well waft in tiny sufficient particles to float right through the fabric.

Homemade masks are not medical equipment and as surgical masks and respirators are not governed. Their usage presents a range of restrictions:

- They have not been checked in compliance with recognized guidelines,

- The materials are not the same as those used in surgical masks or respirators,

- The ridges of which are not devised to form a barrier around the nose and mouth that may not offer full protection from virus-sized particles

- That can be hard to breathe and may stop you from getting the reaction

www.ingramcontent.com/pod-product-compliance
Lightning Source LLC
Chambersburg PA
CBHW050001230526
45465CB00003BB/1206